Pharmacology – Research, Safety Testing and Regulation

THE PHARMACOLOGICAL GUIDE TO MONTELUKAST

PHARMACOLOGY – RESEARCH, SAFETY TESTING AND REGULATION

Additional books and e-books in this series can be found on Nova's website under the Series tab.

Pharmacology – Research, Safety Testing and Regulation

The Pharmacological Guide to Montelukast

Søren C. Dam
Editor

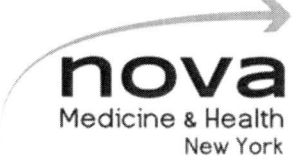

Copyright © 2019 by Nova Science Publishers, Inc.

All rights reserved. No part of this book may be reproduced, stored in a retrieval system or transmitted in any form or by any means: electronic, electrostatic, magnetic, tape, mechanical photocopying, recording or otherwise without the written permission of the Publisher.

We have partnered with Copyright Clearance Center to make it easy for you to obtain permissions to reuse content from this publication. Simply navigate to this **publication**'s page on Nova's website and locate the "Get Permission" button below the title description. This button is linked directly to the title's permission page on copyright.com. Alternatively, you can visit copyright.com and search by title, ISBN, or ISSN.

For further questions about using the service on copyright.com, please contact:
Copyright Clearance Center
Phone: +1-(978) 750-8400　　　　Fax: +1-(978) 750-4470　　　　E-mail: info@copyright.com.

NOTICE TO THE READER

The Publisher has taken reasonable care in the preparation of this book, but makes no expressed or implied warranty of any kind and assumes no responsibility for any errors or omissions. No liability is assumed for incidental or consequential damages in connection with or arising out of information contained in this book. The Publisher shall not be liable for any special, consequential, or exemplary damages resulting, in whole or in part, from the **readers**' use of, or reliance upon, this material. Any parts of this book based on government reports are so indicated and copyright is claimed for those parts to the extent applicable to compilations of such works.

Independent verification should be sought for any data, advice or recommendations contained in this book. In addition, no responsibility is assumed by the Publisher for any injury and/or damage to persons or property arising from any methods, products, instructions, ideas or otherwise contained in this publication.

This publication is designed to provide accurate and authoritative information with regard to the subject matter covered herein. It is sold with the clear understanding that the Publisher is not engaged in rendering legal or any other professional services. If legal or any other expert assistance is required, the services of a competent person should be sought. FROM A DECLARATION OF PARTICIPANTS JOINTLY ADOPTED BY A COMMITTEE OF THE AMERICAN BAR ASSOCIATION AND A COMMITTEE OF PUBLISHERS.

Additional color graphics may be available in the e-book version of this book.

Library of Congress Cataloging-in-Publication Data

ISBN: 978-1-53616-394-0

Published by Nova Science Publishers, Inc. † New York

CONTENTS

Preface		vii
Chapter 1	Montelukast Encapsulation at the Micro, Nano and Molecular Scale *Susana Santos Braga, Jéssica S. Barbosa and Filipe A. Almeida Paz*	1
Chapter 2	Montelukast as Add-on Therapy to Asthma Treatment Improves Symptom Control and Quality of Life *Fikret Vehbi Izzettin, Esra Yildirim, Birsen Pinar Yildiz, Beyza Torun, Mesut Sancar, Baris Anil and Sule Apikoglu-Rabus*	19
Chapter 3	The Efficacy of Montelukast in the Treatment of Allergic Rhinitis *Cigdem Kalaycik Ertugay and Ela Araz Server*	89
Index		99
Related Nova Publications		105

PREFACE

The Pharmacological Guide to Montelukast opens by presenting the most recent updates on the improvement of montelukast stability and bioavailability, along with some innovative formulations produced by this research. Montelukast is a leukotriene modifier with bronchoprotective and anti-inflammatory actions frequently used in asthma management.

As such, the authors go on to assess the impact of the addition of montelukast to ongoing asthma treatment in terms of improvement in clinical parameters, symptom control and quality of life.

The closing chapter focuses on leukotrienes, formed by leukocytes, which are inflammatory mediators that play an active role in early and late-phase immune response. This group includes montelukast, zafirlukast and prankulast.

Chapter 1 - Montelukast is a leukotriene modifier with bronchoprotective and anti-inflammatory actions frequently used in asthma management. It also has anti-allergic properties, which has lead to a growing popularity and broadened uses. Presently available only as oral solid dosage forms, montelukast use is limited in paediatrics and patients with difficulty in swallowing. These limitations are associated with the high sensitivity of the drug to the combined action of light and humidity. The present chapter reports the most recent updates on the improvement of montelukast stability and bioavailability, along with some innovative formulations produced by this research. Stability can be achieved by protecting montelukast using encapsulation techniques, either at the molecular level using cyclodextrins, or at the micro/nano scale, using polymeric or lipidic particles. The new dosage forms include liquid oral dosage forms and prospect formulations designed for local action at the nasal mucosa, the pulmonary epithelium, or even for targeted delivery at the coronary vascular epithelium.

Chapter 2 - *Introduction*: Asthma like other chronic diseases affects the physical, emotional and social aspects of a patient's life. Thus, the impact of new treatment modalities is needed to be assessed in terms of both clinical and humanistic outcomes. The aim of this study is to assess the impact of addition of montelukast to the ongoing asthma treatment in terms of improvement in clinical parameters, symptom control and quality of life (QOL). *Methods:* The subjects (n=50) consisted of asthma patients aged between 18-65 years, who were not receiving a leukotriene receptor antagonist and who accepted to participate in the study on admittance to the outpatient asthma clinic where the study was conducted. These patients were receiving inhaled corticosteroid (ICS) w/wo long-acting beta2-adrenoceptor agonist (LABA) [+ rapid onset bronchodilator prn] as their maintenance therapies. At the initial visit, the baseline clinical, medication-related and QOL data were recorded and montelukast was added to their therapies. The patients were followed-up for three months and at the final visit, the clinical data as presented by FEV1%, disease severity, symptom control status and the QOL data were recorded again and analyzed for any improvement through the 3-month period. Disease severity was graded according to the Global Initiative for Asthma (GINA) guidelines. Asthma Control Test (ACT) was used in order to assess the symptom control. Asthma Quality of Life Questionnaire (AQLQ) was used to assess the asthma-related QOL of the patients. *Results:* Mean (SEM) age of the patients was 38.6 (1.7) and 80% of the patients was female. The medications used for maintenance asthma treatment other than montelukast were high-dose ICS w/LABA (26%), moderate-dose ICS w/wo LABA (40%/8%) and low-dose ICS w/wo LABA (16%/10%). Addition of montelukast resulted in improvement in disease severity (rate of uncontrolled patients decreased from 86% to 50%, p<0.05); improved symptom control: (median [min-max] ACT score increased from 13 [5-25] to 19.5 [10-25], p<0.001); improved QOL: (median [min-max] AQLQ score increased from 104.5 [45-213] to 156.5 [74-224], p<0.001); while similar improvements were observed for all domains of the AQLQ. The mean (SEM) FEV1 increased from 73.08% (2.1%) to 87.15% (1.6%) at the end of three-months (p<0.001). *Conclusion:* Addition of montelukast to the ongoing asthma treatment resulted in favorable outcomes in terms of improved disease severity, symptom control and QOL.

Chapter 3 - Leukotrienes, formed by leukocytes, are the inflammatory mediators which play an active role both in the early and late-phase immune response. Cysteinyl-leukotriene receptor antagonists are used in the treatment of allergic rhinitis as they inhibit the end-organ response by blocking the leukotriene receptors. This group includes montelukast, zafirlukast and prankulast. Montelukasts are effective on congestion, rhinorrhea, itching and sneezing which compromise the four main daytime symptoms of allergic rhinitis. Antihistaminics and nasal steroids are the main treatment modalities in allergic rhinitis. However, when compared with the placebo, montelukast is more effective on nasal and ocular symptoms. ARIA guideline also proposed montelukast in the seasonal allergic rhinitis of adults and perennial allergic rhinitis of children. Recent studies have mainly focused on combined use of montelukast and antihistaminics and reported that these combinations are as effective as nasal steroids. Further double-blind placebo controlled studies with large study population which evaluates the efficacy of montelukast and also the combined use of montelukasts and antihistaminics should be performed. These studies can provide wider use of montelukast in the treatment of allergic rhinitis.

In: The Pharmacological Guide to Montelukast ISBN: 978-1-53616-394-0
Editor: Søren C. Dam   © 2019 Nova Science Publishers, Inc.

Chapter 1

MONTELUKAST ENCAPSULATION AT THE MICRO, NANO AND MOLECULAR SCALE

Susana Santos Braga[1,*], Jéssica S. Barbosa[1,2] and Filipe A. Almeida Paz[2,]

[1] QOPNA & LAQV-REQUIMTE, Department of Chemistry, University of Aveiro, Aveiro, Portugal
[2] CICECO - Aveiro Institute of Materials, Department of Chemistry, University of Aveiro, Aveiro, Portugal

ABSTRACT

Montelukast is a leukotriene modifier with bronchoprotective and anti-inflammatory actions frequently used in asthma management. It also has anti-allergic properties, which has lead to a growing popularity and broadened uses. Presently available only as oral solid dosage forms, montelukast use is limited in paediatrics and patients with difficulty in

---

* Corresponding Author`s E-mail: sbraga@ua.pt.

swallowing. These limitations are associated with the high sensitivity of the drug to the combined action of light and humidity.

The present chapter reports the most recent updates on the improvement of montelukast stability and bioavailability, along with some innovative formulations produced by this research. Stability can be achieved by protecting montelukast using encapsulation techniques, either at the molecular level using cyclodextrins, or at the micro/nano scale, using polymeric or lipidic particles. The new dosage forms include liquid oral dosage forms and prospect formulations designed for local action at the nasal mucosa, the pulmonary epithelium, or even for targeted delivery at the coronary vascular epithelium.

Keywords: drug delivery, drug dosage forms, nanoparticles, microparticles, cyclodextrins

ABBREVIATIONS

CD,	cyclodextrin
CysLT,	cystenyl leukotriene
$CysLTR_1$,	cystenyl leukotriene receptor type 1
EMA,	European Medicines Agency
FDA,	U.S. Food and Drug Administration
NLC,	nanostructured lipid carrier
NP,	nanoparticle
PLA,	poly-lactic acid
RH,	relative humidity
SLN,	solid lipid nanoparticle

INTRODUCTION

Montelukast is used by millions of asthma and allegy patients around the world, with market sales of over 700 million US dollars yearly for the Singulair brand alone [1]. Montelukast was developed as part of a program designed to obtain 'leukotriene modifiers', molecules able to block or modify the effect of leukotrienes by stopping them from binding to their receptors, and it was the best of its class [2]. The leukotriene receptors (CysLTR$_1$) targeted by montelukast mediate the pathophysiological alterations occuring during asthma, namely inflammation, broncoconstriction and the production of mucus. Today, cystenyl leucotrienes (CysLTs) are also known to be involved in various allergic responses, including mucus production and inflammatory cell migration in allergic rhinitis, skin fibrosis and collagen deposition in atopic dermatitis, allergic conjunctivitis and even some anaphylatic reactions [3]. This way, montelukast, by interfering with CysLTs, has also anti-allergic activity. Nowadays, it is employed to prevent and treat seasonal allergies and a much broader set of immune disfunctions that go far beyond its classical asthma regulating role.

CURRENT MONTELUKAST FORMULATIONS

Montelukast is a neutral molecule, with the structure corresponding to the two-dimensional representation in Figure 1. In its original neutral form, montelukast solubility in water is quite low, rounding 0.2-0.5 µg/mL at 25ºC. The formation of a sodium salt at the carboxylic group allows increasing the overall solubility to 100-1000 µg/mL.

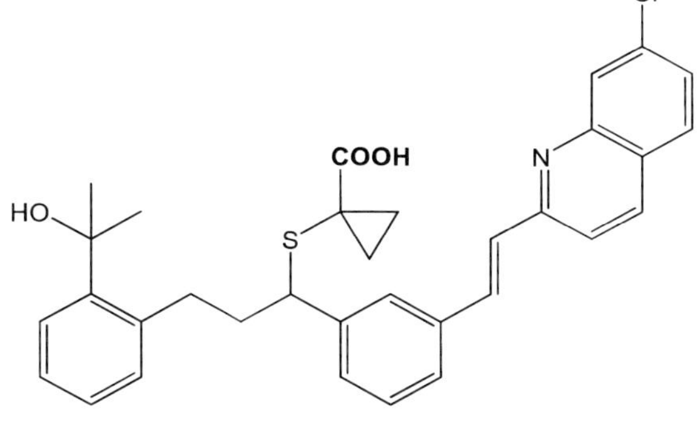

Figure 1. Structural representation of montelukast; the carboxyl is highlighted in bold.

The sodium salt is the commercialized form of this drug. Presently, montelukast sodium (hereafter called as montelukast, for simplicity) is available from many pharmaceutical companies, either under the tradename Singulair® (by Merk) or as a generic. All marketed formulations are solid dosage forms, and these include tablets, chewable tablets and oral granules (Table 1).

Table 1. Doses and recommendations for use of the montelukast formulations currently available in the market

Formulation	Dose	Applications and advantages	Target age group
oral granules	4 mg	Easy to swallow Compatible with water, lactant's milk and a few soft foods (apple sauce, carrot, rice, ice-cream)	6 months - 5 years
chewable tablets	4 mg	Suitable for young children[a,b]	2 - 5 years
chewable tablets	5 mg	Suitable for youngsters[a,b]	6 - 14 years
film-coated tablets	10 mg	Resistant to daylight[a,b]	≥15 years

[a] From Storms et al. [4] [b] from Al Omari et al. [5].

The fact that the dosage forms currently available are all solid products is related to the limitations imposed by montelukast, a compound sensitive to light, temperature, humidity and oxidation [5-7]. The lack of liquid formulations makes administration of montelukast to small babies a quite challenging process. The only product available is a granulate that is compatible with water, with milk (from the mother or lactant formulas) and a with short list of soft foods, namely applesauce, carrots, rice, or ice cream, but requires administration within the next 15 minutes after dispersion into the medium [8].

The chewable tablets, recommended for young children, are also problematic because many brands (including Singulair) and generics contain the sweetener aspartame. This makes them unsuited for patients with phenylketonuria [8].

Pharmacokinetics, Interactions, and Adverse Reactions

Montelukast levels in the blood after oral intake correspond to approximately 61-73% of the amount taken by the patient, mainly due to losses during gastroenteric absorption that are influenced by the presence or absence of food, and to the effect of hepatic first pass metabolism [9]. Montelukast is extensively oxidized in the liver by the cytochrome P450 enzyme system, being subsequently excreted into the bile [9, 10]. Thus, its permanence in the bloodstream is relatively short, with a peak around 2 to 4 h after intake and a half-life of 2.7 to 5.5 h [11].

Montelukast is generally well tolerated and adverse reactions are rare. These have higher incidence in infants and manifest mostly as neurological or mood alterations such as an increased aggressive behaviour and the occurrence of nightmares [12]. In adults, headache is the most reported adverse effect [12], followed by hypersensitivity cases that may result in autoimmune vasculitis, or, in extreme situations, in anaphylaxis [13]. There is also a single case report of montelukast interaction with corticosteroids which led to the retention of fluids in the patient and a severe peripheral edema (with 13 Kg weight gain) [14]. This was resolved upon discontinuation of the corticosteroid while maintaining treatment with montelukast.

Interactions of montelukast with other drugs may have different effects. Its plasma concentration may be reduced by up to 40% due to interaction with phenobarbital [8]. In turn, plasma concentration of montelukast may be exceedingly increased upon interaction with drugs that block the main enzyme responsible for its metabolism, CYP2C8, such as gemfibrozil [15].

NANO AND MOLECULAR ENCAPSULATION OF MONTELUKAST

In the last decade, several studies have reported new encapsulation strategies for montelukast, at the nano and molecular scales. These aim at improving the stability and, in a few instances, serve as the starting ground for alternative routes of delivery.

Polymeric Nanoparticles

Encapsulation of montelukast into chitosan nanoparticles (NPs) was reported by Inamdar *et al.* to allow a sustained delivery by inhalation. Chitosan NPs loaded with montelukast are deposited on the lungs and the drug is slowly absorbed over a period of 24 h [16]. As a comment on this report, we note that, while the use of chitosan as a carrier brings advantages for pulmonar delivery due to its mucoadhesive properties [17], chitosan-based nanotechnologies are still far from reaching the market. Indeed, chitosan is not approved by the FDA and toxicologic data on humans is lacking; in zebrafish, chitosan-NPs are known to be toxic [18]. Moreover, chitosan may work as an immunogenic agent [17], which is conter-productive in a scenario of asthma. Alternatively, montelukast can be encapsulated into particles made from the FDA-approved poly-lactic acid (PLA) carrier [19]. Although their particle size is too large to consider them as nanoparticles, the PLA carriers containing montelukast were shown to outperform conventional oral dosage forms in reducing airway inflamation in asthmatic mice.

Lipid-Based Nanoparticles

Encapsulation of montelukast into lipid-based nanoparticles is reported by various research groups. Made from physiological lipids, these NPs have a series of advantages over the ones made from polymers. Not only are they biocompatible and fully biodegradable, thus eliminating toxicity associated with *in vivo* degradation of polymers, as they improve bioavailability by promoting oral absorption via selective lymphatic uptake [20, 21].

One class of lipid nanoparticles comprises the so-called SLNs, acronym for 'solid lipid nanoparticles', although the material is not really a solid but rather a super-cooled mixed phase, that is, it contains some lipid crystals and a few crystals of guest drug. These materials are somewhat instable since lipids tend to revert to the lower-energy liquid form over time. Nevertheless, encapsulation of montelukast into SLNs allowed forming a stable product that lasts up to 30 days in storage [22].

A second generation of lipid nanoparticles, called NLCs from 'nanostructured lipid carriers', was shown to encapsulate montelukast with a very high loading efficacy (96.1%) and to increase its oral bioavailability in Wistar rats by 143-fold while maintaining a sustained release profile of $c.a.$ 24 h [21]. Aiming at controlled pulmonary delivery, the same montelukast-loaded NLCs were tested in simulated lung fluid, demonstrating drug release in a sustained manner: 60% of the drug is released in a quasi linear time-dose plot over the first 12 h while the remaining drug load takes over 24 h to be fully released [23].

Molecular Capsules

Molecular encapsulation of montelukast can be achieved with cyclodextrins, naturally occuring cyclic oligomers of 1,4-linked α-D-glucose [24, 25]. Native cyclodextrins typically have six to eight units, being coined as α-CD, β-CD and γ-CD, and they are approved for human use by the FDA, both in pharmaceutical and in food applications [26]. A few chemically modified derivatives, with highlight to hydroxypropyl-β-CD (HPβCD), are also FDA-approved for pharmaceutical use. Inclusion of a drug into the ring cavity of a cyclodextrin occurs by Van der Waals and hydrophobic interactions with the apolar fragments of the drug to form the so-called inclusion complexes. With montelukast, true inclusion was demonstrated to be achieved only using γ-CD, since the cavity sizes of the hosts α-CD and β-CD are too small to accommodate the large molecules of this drug. Furthermore, it was demonstrated that the inclusion complexation can be done by solid-solid interactions under a co-milling process [27]. This process is highly advantageous for a water-sensitive drug such as monteluakst because it eliminates the need of solvents. Inclusion of montelukast into γ-CD was further shown to improve its stability: when the complex is dissolved in water, drug concentrations remain stable for at least 4 h, but when the pure drug is dissolved its concentration drops after 30 to 60 min [27]. A possible application of the γ-CD·montelukast inclusion complex would be as part of a dispersible powder or granulate with longer stability following preparation (we recall that the currently marketed formulation is only stable for 15 min).

ENCAPSULATION-BASED NEW DOSAGE FORMS

Liquid Formulations

The lack of montelukast liquid formulations in the market has driven research efforts to find solutions on how to achieve them. Such solutions must obviously include adequate solubilizers, as well as strong stabilizers, to ensure montelukast is not degraded while in an aqueous medium – the most challenging step. Of the different methodologies presented in the literature for these two requirements, molecular encapsulation with resource to cyclodextrins is the most practical one, since it allows the simultaneous fulfillment of both. Alternatively, micro- or nano-encapsulation procedures are also available.

Inclusion of montelukast into lipidic nanodroplets to form a nanoemulsion in water was recently proposed by Almajidi *et al*. The nanoemulsion is optically clear due to the small size of the droplets and it contains also orange flavor for better taste, being presented by the authors as a stable, easy-to-swallow oral dosage form for montelukast [28].

A clear aqueous solution of montelukast featuring good stability and being bioequivalent to the granules currently employed for administration to babies is reported by Kim et al. The oral solution contains montelukast sodium, HPβCD, methylparaben sodium, propylparaben sodium and EDTA sodium at w/v percentages of 1.04/156/1.8/0.2/1. The *in vitro* dissolution profile in the FDA-regulated medium is equivalent to that of the granules, and *in vivo* studies show similar plasma concentrations and pharmacokinetic parameters to the commercial granules, suggesting that it was bioequivalent to these in rats. Moreover, it is physically and chemically stable for at least 12 months at 25 °C with 60% RH and 40 °C with 75% RH. The authors have thus recommended their newly-developed solution as a strong alternative to the granules for the treatment of asthma [29].

A liquid formulation for montelukast claimed to feature 'superior stability, taste and flavor' is patented by Kwon *et al.* The drug is solubilized with the help of native cyclodextrins or by a water-soluble polymer, and the formulation further comprises a sweetening agent, a flavoring agent, a preservative, an emulsifier, a coloring agent and a stabilizer [30]. It should be noted that the amount of cyclodextrins employed in the formulations covered by this patent is very high, in a large excess to the amount of montelukast. The CD-to-montelukast ratio varies between 40:1 and 200:1 [30], which explains why cyclodextrins with smaller cavities such as α-CD and β-CD can still solubilize the drug: the presence of large excess of host molecules allows multiple interactions of the non-inclusion type with fragments of montelukast molecules, and these favour solubilization.

A set of formulations for nasal delivery with two active ingredients, the anti-histamine loratadine and montelukast is patented by Bhattacharya *et al.* The formulations are water-based and they can be presented as a variety of fluids, ranging from solutions to gels; their composition further comprises solubilizers (alcohol or polyols), polymeric thickening/dispersing agents, emulsifiers, surfactants, and antioxidants or cyclodextrins as stabilizers. The cyclodextrins patented for use in these formulations may be either γ-CD or HPβCD, and their stabilizing action is attributed to the formation of inclusion complexes [31].

An uncommon family of cyclodextrin derivatives – hydroxybutenyl cyclodextrins – are also patented as solubilizers for a large variety of drugs, in which montelukast is included [32]. The patent also includes compositions of solutions containing the drug and the cyclodextrin, which comprise mainly an organic, water-miscible solvent, and a small amount of water (mass percentage of 10% or less). The hydroxybutenyl cyclodextrins are claimed to increase the solubility of the target drugs by formation of inclusion complexes. As a note to this patent on new cyclodextrin derivatives for use as solubilizers, it should be noted that new chemical entities, even when designed to be used merely as functional excipients, require approval by regulatory entities such as the DFA and the EMA before human use, thus meaning that hydroxybutenyl cyclodextrins, not yet approved by these agencies, are still very far from reaching the market.

Solid Formulations

A handful of innovative solid dosage forms based on cyclodextrins are also known. In these formulations, it is difficult to verify that cyclodextrins are forming true inclusion complexes with montelukast; nevertheless, their presence contributes to the stabilization of the drug.

Montelukast granules containing calcium citrate as a combination therapeutic agent are patented by Mei *et al*. Besides the active ingredients, the granules are comprised by HPβCD, sweeteners (stevia and/or aspartame) and sodium hydroxypropyl starch. Claimed uses of the granules are in the treatment of asthma and allergic rhinitis [33].

Other granules featuring montelukast, either alone or in combination with the anti-histamine drug levocetirizine, are patented by Im *et al*. The granules are claimed to have increased stability and bioavailability, but also to improve patient compliance owing to the effective masking of bitter taste [34]. The superior performance of the granules over the currently available formulations is attributed to the use of cyclodextrins in the formula, particularly β-CD or HPβCD. In another patent on montelukast/levocetirizine mixed granules, HPβCD is used in small amounts with the purpose of acting not as a stabilizing molecular capsule but rather as a binding agent, that is, a material that helps hold the particles of the granulate together; instead, meglumine is used as stabilizer [35].

A recent trend in montelukast solid oral dosage forms is the chronotherapeutic approach [36, 37]. In this method, the dosage form allows the drug to be available for absorption at a prescribed time, according to the circadian rhythm of the pathology, optimizing the therapeutic outcome and minimizing side effects. The latest developments in chronotherapeutic oral dosage forms for montelukast, reported by Lavakumar *et al.* in 2018, use microencapsulation as a strategy to achieve the specific drug delivery goals. Montelukast is encapsulated into polymeric microcapsules (made from a commercial polymer, Eudragit) and these microcapsules are inserted into a larger hydrogel capsule (made of kondagogu gum) that is resistant to gastric and small intestine media and designed to release the microcapsules five hours after ingestion; then, the free microcapsules release montelukast drug over a 16 hour period [38]. When taken around 11 p.m., these dosage forms may help avoid nocturnal asthma surges, which occur typically from 4 to 6 a.m., and the sustained release profile will further assist the patient during most of the daytime.

NEW THERAPEUTIC APPLICATIONS OF ENCAPSULATED MONTELUKAST

The anti-inflammatory properties of monteluksat make it a drug with a large potential of applications. To use montelukast beyond the currently approved scenarios of asthma and allergy management, targeted drug delivery strategies are under study. These rely on the encapsulation of montelukast into functional nanoparticles that can be directed to a specific target of the patient. An example of this application involves the study of montelukast as a post-operatory treatment to avoid restenosis in coronary arteries subject to stent cirgury. Collapsed coronary arteries are treated with stents to maintain the flow of blood to the cardiac tissue, however, following the surgical intervention, inflammatory response in the surrounding vessel wall often causes the blood vessel walls to thicken and eventually clog once more. Targeting an anti-inflammatory agent towards this site is a innovative strategy to prevent such complications. Montelukast was loaded into rosin gum nanoparticles, containing also smaller magnetic nanoparticles and a chondroitin coating [39]. The coating allows the nanoparticles to adhere to entothelial vascular cells, providing the first level of targeted delivery; targeting is further complemented by the presence of the magnetic nanoparticles, which will allow the nanoparticles to accumulate in the tissue of the patient where a magnetic field is applied. Significant supression of inflammation by action of the montelukast-loaded nanoparticles was demonstrated *in vitro* on cultured human umbilical vein endothelial cells (HUVEC cell line) [39]. Although *in vivo* data is still missing, these promising results open way for a new clinical field of application of nanoparticle-encapsulated montelukast.

CONCLUSION

This chapter describes the limitations of the currently available dosage forms of montelukast, along with the underlying physico-chemical properties, and presents the results of the most recent research efforts in finding improved formulations, alternative routes of delivery and new clinical applications that will expand the use of this drug.

Highlight must be given to liquid oral dosage forms which are, as mentioned previously, current unavailable in the market and thus the most soughtafter formulations. Recent literature reports features two different encapsulation-based approaches for obtaining them, one using nanodroplets to encapsulate montelukast and another using CDs as molecular capsules. The lipidic nanodroplets approach has the benefit of providing a transparent nanoemulsion [28] at a low cost, while the formulations based on molecular encapsulation [29, 30] require a very large amount of CDs to afford the desired performance and thus they are expected to be expensive products due to relatively high price of CDs.

Noteworthy is also the use of the stabilization properties of CDs to obtain innovative dosage forms combining montelukast with other drugs, such as anti-histamin agents and calcium citrate. Within these, highlight goes to the dosage forms designed for local action at the nasal mucosa [31]. These offer not only a new application site for montelukast but also the possibility of affordable new products, because no large amounts of CDs are required in their composition.

A final word goes to the expansion of therapeutic applications of montelukast that is expected to arise as a consequence of the discovery of $CysLTR_1$ in tissues beyong the bronchial smooth muscle and nasal mucosa, namely blood cells and vascular endothelial cells [40]. Once more, encapsulation of montelukast is crucial to achieve funtional formulations with clinical application in new fields, as demonstrated by the example of magnetic-directed nanoparticles to deliver montelukast to the endothelium of coronary arteries [39].

ACKNOWLEDGMENTS

Thanks are due to the University of Aveiro and FCT/MCT (Fundação para a Ciência e Tecnologia, Ministério da Educação e da Ciência) for financial support to the QOPNA research Unit (FCT Ref UID/QUI/00062/2019) and to the project CICECO – Aveiro Institute of Materials (FCT Ref. UID/CTM/50011/2019) through national founds and, where applicable, co-financed by the FEDER (European Fund for Regional Development), within the PT2020 Partnership Agreement. JSB gratefully acknowledges FCT for the Ph.D. grant No. PD/BD/135104/2017.

REFERENCES

[1] Merk, Sharp and Dohme Corp. *Merck Announces Fourth-Quarter and Full-Year 2018 Financial Results*. Press release of 1st February 2019. https:// investors.merck.com/ news/press-release-details/ 2019/ Merck- Announces- Fourth- Quarter- and- Full- Year- 2018- Financial-Results/default.aspx [last accessed on 10 April, 2019].

[2] Young, R. N. (2001) The discovery of montelukast (Singulair): a leukotriene receptor antagonist for the treatment of asthma. *Séminaires & Conférences Chimie École Doctorale 459*, 29 September, Université de Montpellier II, Montpellier. France.

[3] Liu, M. and Yokomizo, T. (2015) The role of leukotrienes in allergic diseases, *Allergol Int*, 64: 17–26.

[4] Storms, W., Michele, T. M., Knorr, B., Noonan, G., Shapiro, G., Zhang, J., Shingo, S. and Reiss, T. F. (2001). Clinical safety and tolerability of montelukast, a leukotriene receptor antagonist, in controlled clinical trials in patients aged >= 6 years. *Clin Exp Allergy*, 31: 77–87.

[5] Al Omari, M. M., Zoubi, R. M., Hasan, E. I., Khader, T. Z. and Badwan, A. A. (2007). Effect of light and heat on the stability of montelukast in solution and in its solid state. *J Pharm Biomed Anal*, 45: 465–471.

[6] Okumu, A., DiMaso, M. and Lobenberg, R. (2008). Dynamic Dissolution Testing To Establish In Vitro/In Vivo Correlations for Montelukast Sodium, a Poorly Soluble Drug. *Pharm Res*, 25: 2778–85.

[7] Rashmitha, N., Raj, T. J. S., Srinivas, C., Srinivas, N., Ray, U. K., Sharma, Hemant Kumar and Mukkanti, K. (2010). A Validated RP-HPLC Method for the Determination of Impurities in Montelukast Sodium. *E-J Chem*, 7: 555–563.

[8] Merck Sharp & Dohme Corp (1998-2019). *Prescribing Information for Singulair.* https://www.merck.com/product/usa/pi_circulars/s/singulair/singulair_pi.pdf [last accessed on 11 April, 2019].

[9] Cheng, H. Leff, J. A. Amin, R., Gertz, B. J., De Smet, M., Noonan, N., Rogers, J. D., Malbecq, W., Meisner, D. and Somers, G. (1996). Pharmacokinetics, bioavailability, and safety of montelukast sodium (MK-0476) in healthy males and females. *Pharmaceut Res*, 13: 445–448.

[10] Filppula, A. M., Laitila, J., Neuvonen, P.J. and Backman, J.T. (2011). Reevaluation of the microsomal metabolism of montelukast: major

contribution by CYP2C8 at clinically relevant concentrations. *Drug Metab Dispos*, 39: 904–911.

[11] Kearns, G. L., Lu, S. S., Maganti, L., Li, X. S., Migoya, E., Ahmed, T., Knorr, B. and Reiss, T. F. (2008). Pharmacokinetics and safety of montelukast oral granules in children 1 to 3 months of age with bronchiolitis. *J Clin Pharmacol*, 48: 502–511.

[12] Haarman, M. G., van Hunsel, F. and de Vries, T. W. (2017). Adverse drug reactions of montelukast in children and adults. *Pharma Res Per*, 5: e00341.

[13] Calapai, G., Casciaro, M., Miroddi, M., Calapai, F., Navarra, M. and Gangemi, S. (2014). Montelukast-Induced Adverse Drug Reactions: A Review of Case Reports in the Literature. *Pharmacology* 94: 60–70.

[14] Geller, M. (2000). Marked peripheral edema associated with montelukast and prednisolone. *Am Intern Med*, 132: 924.

[15] Karonen, T., Filppula, A., Laitila, J., Niemi, M., Neuvonen, P. J. and Backman, J. T. (2010). Gemfibrozil markedly increases the plasma concentrations of montelukast: a previously unrecognized role for CYP2C8 in the metabolism of montelukast. *Clin Pharmacol Ther*, 88: 223–230.

[16] Inamdar, B. P., Kathawala, K. J., Parikh, A. Y., Shah, T. R., Shah, J. N. (2013). Formulation, development and characterization of chitosan nanoparticles of montelukast sodium for site specific drug delivery in management of asthma. *Int J Drug Formulation Res* 4: 87–101.

[17] Islam, N., Ferro, V., (2016). Recent Advances in Chitosan-Based Nanoparticulate Pulmonary Drug Delivery. *Nanoscale* 8: 14341–14358.

[18] Hu, Y. L., Qi, W., Han, F., Shao, J. Z., Gao, J. Q. (2011). Toxicity evaluation of biodegradable chitosan nanoparticles using a zebrafish embryo model. *Int J Nanomed* 6: 3351–3359.

[19] Patel, B., Gupta, N., Ahsan, F. (2014). Aerosolized Montelukast Polymeric Particles - An Alternative to Oral Montelukast-Alleviate Symptoms of Asthma in a Rodent Model. *Pharm Res* 31: 3095–3105.

[20] Das, S., Chaudhury, A. (2011). Recent Advances in Lipid Nanoparticle Formulations with Solid Matrix for Oral Drug Delivery. *AAPS Pharm Sci Tech* 12: 62–76.

[21] Patil-Gadhe, A., Pokharkar, V. (2014). Montelukast-loaded nanostructured lipid carriers: Part I Oral bioavailability improvement. *Eur J Pharm Biopharm* 88: 160–168.

[22] Priyanka, K., Sathali, A. A. H. (2012). Preparation and Evaluation of Montelukast Sodium Loaded Solid Lipid Nanoparticles. *J Young Pharm* 4: 129–137.

[23] Patil-Gadhe, A., Kyadarkunte, A., Patole, M., Pokharkar, V. (2014). Montelukast-loaded nanostructured lipid carriers: Part II Pulmonary drug delivery and in vitro–in vivo aerosol performance. *Eur J Pharm Biopharm* 88: 169–177.

[24] Villiers, A. (1891). Sur la fermentation de la fécule par l'action du ferment butyrique. *Compt Rend Acad Sci* 112: 536–538. [On the fermentation of starch by the action of butyric ferment. *Compt Rend Acad Sci* 112: 536–538]

[25] Schardinger, F. (1903). Über thermophile Bakterien aus versehiedenen Speisen and Milch [About thermophilic bacteria from food and milk]. *Z Unters Nahr u Genussm* 6: 865–880.

[26] Pereira, A. B., Braga, S. S. In *Cyclodextrins: Synthesis, Chemical Applications and Role in Drug Delivery*; Ramirez, F. G., Ed, Novascience publishers: Hauppauge, NY, 2015, Chapter 6: 195–224.

[27] Barbosa, J. S., Nolasco, M, Ribeiro-Claro, P., Paz, F. A. A., Braga, S. S. (2019). Pre-formulation studies of the γ-cyclodextrin and montelukast inclusion compound prepared by co-milling. *J Pharm Sci* 108:1837–1847.

[28] Almajidi, Y. Q., Mahdi, Z. H., Maraie, N. K. (2018). Preparation and in vitro evaluation of montelukast sodium oral nanoemulsion. *Int J Appl Pharm*, 10: 49–53.

[29] Kim, Y. H., Kim, D. K., Kwon, M. S., Kwon, T. K., Park, J. H., Jin, S. G., Kim, K. S., Kim, Y. I., Park, J.-H., Kim, J. O., Yong, C. S., Woo, J. S., Choi, H.-G. (2015). Novel montelukast sodium-loaded clear oral solution prepared with hydroxypropyl-β-cyclodextrin as a

solubilizer and stabilizer: enhanced stability and bioequivalence to commercial granules in rats. *J Inclus Phen Macro Chem*, 82: 479–487.

[30] Kwon, T. K., Choi, Y. K., Yan, X. W., Wang, Z. Z., Kim, Y. L., Park, J. H., Woo, J. S. (2015). *Liquid formulation comprising montelukast or pharmaceutically acceptable salt thereof and method for preparing same.* Patent WO2015093847A1, July 25th.

[31] Bhattacharya, S., Chhabada, S., Lagu, K. (2003) *Intranasal pharmaceutical compositions comprising an antihistamine and a leukotriene inhibitor.* Patent WO2003101434 A2, Dec 11th.

[32] Buchanan, C., Buchanan, N., Lambert, J., Posey-Dowty, J. (2004). *Cyclodextrin solubilizers for liquid and semi-solid formulations.* Patent US20060105045A1, Nov 8th.

[33] Mei, Y., Luo, L., He, y., Ma, G., Jiang, Y., Yang, L., Chen, L., Li, X. (2012) *Montelukast sodium combination drug granules for treating asthma, and application thereof.* Patent CN102688238 (A), June 18th.

[34] Im, H. T., Kim, Y. I., Park, J. H., Woo, J. S., Kwon, T. K. (2014). *Complex granule formulation having improved stability comprising levocetirizine and montelukast.* Patent WO 2014208915A3, Dec 31st.

[35] Yan, X., Yang, H. (2015) *Particle composition, preparation method and formulation therefor.* Patent WO2015062466 A1, May 7th.

[36] Padmaxi, B., Karwa, P., Patel, K., Sahidullah, M. M., Irshad, P. M. (2012). Formulation and evaluation of time controlled drug delivery system of Montelukast sodium. *Int J Pharm Innovations* 2:1–12.

[37] Ranjan, O. P., Nayak, U. Y., Reddy, M. S., Dengale, S. J., Musmade, P. B., Udupa, N. (2014). Osmotically controlled pulsatile release capsule of montelukast sodium for chronotherapy: Statistical optimization, *in vitro* and *in vivo* evaluation. *Drug deliv* 21: 509–518.

[38] Lavakumar, V., Sowmya1, C., Venkateshan, N., Ravichandiran, V., Leela, K. V., Harikrishanan, N., Anbu, J. (2018). Microcapsule‑based chronomodulated drug delivery systems of montelukast sodium in the treatment of nocturnal asthma. *Int J Pharm Invest* 8: 24–32.

[39] Varshosaz, J., Javanmard, S. H., Soghratia, S., Behdadfarc, B. (2016). Magnetic chondroitin targeted nanoparticles for dual targeting of montelukast in prevention of in-stent restenosis. *RSC Adv* 6: 12337–12347.
[40] Singh, R. K., Tandon, R., Dastidar, S. G., Ray, A. (2013). A review on leukotrienes and their receptors with reference to asthma. *J Asthma* 50: 922–931.

In: The Pharmacological Guide to Montelukast   ISBN: 978-1-53616-394-0
Editor: Søren C. Dam   © 2019 Nova Science Publishers, Inc.

Chapter 2

MONTELUKAST AS ADD-ON THERAPY TO ASTHMA TREATMENT IMPROVES SYMPTOM CONTROL AND QUALITY OF LIFE

Fikret Vehbi Izzettin[1], PhD, Esra Yildirim[2],
Birsen Pinar Yildiz[3], PhD, Beyza Torun[2],
Mesut Sancar[2], PhD, Baris Anil[3], PhD
and Sule Apikoglu-Rabus[2],*, PhD

[1]Clinical Pharmacy Department, Bezmialem University
Faculty of Pharmacy, Istanbul, Turkey
[2]Clinical Pharmacy Department, Marmara University
Faculty of Pharmacy, Istanbul, Turkey
[3]Pulmonology Department, University of Health Sciences,
Yedikule Training and Research Hospital for
Chest Diseases and Thoracic Surgery, Istanbul, Turkey

---

* Corresponding Author's E-mail: sule.rabus@marmara.edu.tr; sulerabus@yahoo.com.

ABSTRACT

Introduction: Asthma like other chronic diseases affects the physical, emotional and social aspects of a patient's life. Thus, the impact of new treatment modalities is needed to be assessed in terms of both clinical and humanistic outcomes. The aim of this study is to assess the impact of addition of montelukast to the ongoing asthma treatment in terms of improvement in clinical parameters, symptom control and quality of life (QOL).

Methods: The subjects (n=50) consisted of asthma patients aged between 18-65 years, who were not receiving a leukotriene receptor antagonist and who accepted to participate in the study on admittance to the outpatient asthma clinic where the study was conducted. These patients were receiving inhaled corticosteroid (ICS) w/wo long-acting beta2-adrenoceptor agonist (LABA) [+ rapid onset bronchodilator prn] as their maintenance therapies. At the initial visit, the baseline clinical, medication-related and QOL data were recorded and montelukast was added to their therapies. The patients were followed-up for three months and at the final visit, the clinical data as presented by FEV1%, disease severity, symptom control status and the QOL data were recorded again and analyzed for any improvement through the 3-month period. Disease severity was graded according to the Global Initiative for Asthma (GINA) guidelines. Asthma Control Test (ACT) was used in order to assess the symptom control. Asthma Quality of Life Questionnaire (AQLQ) was used to assess the asthma-related QOL of the patients.

Results: Mean (SEM) age of the patients was 38.6 (1.7) and 80% of the patients was female. The medications used for maintenance asthma treatment other than montelukast were high-dose ICS w/LABA (26%), moderate-dose ICS w/wo LABA (40%/8%) and low-dose ICS w/wo LABA (16%/10%). Addition of montelukast resulted in improvement in disease severity (rate of uncontrolled patients decreased from 86% to 50%, $p<0.05$); improved symptom control: (median [min-max] ACT score increased from 13 [5-25] to 19.5 [10-25], $p<0.001$); improved QOL: (median [min-max] AQLQ score increased from 104.5 [45-213] to 156.5 [74-224], $p<0.001$); while similar improvements were observed for all domains of the AQLQ. The mean (SEM) FEV1 increased from 73.08% (2.1%) to 87.15% (1.6%) at the end of three-months ($p<0.001$).

Conclusion: Addition of montelukast to the ongoing asthma treatment resulted in favorable outcomes in terms of improved disease severity, symptom control and QOL.

Keywords: asthma, symptom control, montelukast, quality of life, AQLQ, ACT

1. INTRODUCTION

Asthma is a chronic inflammatory disease that causes wheezing, chest tightness, respiratory distress and cough especially at night and in the early morning. The chronic inflammation causes hyperreactivity in the bronchia and leads to restriction of airflow on exposure to various risk factors [1].

Asthma is a common disease that affects all age groups. In addition to genetic factors, environmental factors play a role in asthma development. Therefore, the frequency of asthma may vary significantly by countries and even regions. In the United States (US), it is estimated that more than 26 million people are suffering from asthma. It is the most common chronic disease among children in the United States, with about 6 million children affected. According to the Centers for Disease Control and Prevention (CDC), it was observed that among asthma patients 11 million were treated as outpatients, 1.7 million were admitted to the emergency room and 439 435 were hospitalized [2-4]. The estimated cost of direct and indirect expenditure related to asthma in the US was $56 billion in 2011 [5].

The economic burden of asthma with its increasing prevalence, morbidity, and mortality had been widely discussed since the second half of the twentieth century. Studies performed in the same society 40 years apart, using standardized methods revealed increases in asthma prevalence. The increase was seen in countries with different lifestyles. It was seen that especially the increase in urban areas with western lifestyle was higher. It was estimated that in 2025, 100 million people would be added to the number of asthma patients recorded in 2001 [6].

In recent years, quality of life measurements are getting increasingly important for the assessment of the treatment of chronic diseases such as asthma, which is affecting the life physically, emotionally and socially, causing loss of productivity and quality of life [7].

Despite the increasing understanding of its physiopathology and the development of effective anti-asthma drugs, mortality and morbidity rates of asthma are increasing all over the world [8].

Asthma is defined by airway inflammation, restriction of respiratory function, and symptoms. For this reason, all these variables are expected to be improved in asthma control. The presence and level of symptoms, decrease in pulmonary function parameters, daily bronchodilator drug needs to relieve symptoms, and activity limitations are checked to determine the level of asthma control. In a fully controlled patient, there should be no day or night symptoms, activity restriction and need for symptom relief medication, while respiratory function parameters (PEF, FEV1) should be within normal limits, and the patient should not have any attacks [9]. The main purpose of asthma treatment is to control the disease by reducing symptoms and attacks and by improving respiratory function [8]. In our study, we determined the level of asthma control by the Asthma Control Test (ACT) as well as according to the Global Initiative for Asthma (GINA) guidelines criteria.

Although the main approach to asthma control is pharmacologic treatment, non-pharmacological measures are also important [10]. As a part of the self-care of the patients, patient monitoring and education are essential throughout the treatment [11].

The leukotriene receptor antagonists zafirlukast and montelukast, and the leukotriene synthesis inhibitor zileuton have been used in children and adults with persistent asthma in the United States since 1996 [12]. Montelukast is used more frequently in asthma maintenance treatment [13].

In this study, we aimed to assess the impact of addition of montelukast to the ongoing asthma treatment in terms of improvement in clinical parameters (i.e., FEV% value), symptom control (based on ACT and GINA criteria) and quality of life (assessed by Asthma Quality of Life Questionnaire).

2. Literature Review

2.1. Asthma

2.1.1. Definition

Asthma is a disease characterized by reversible airflow obstruction and recurrent respiratory symptoms such as shortness of breath, wheezing, chest tightness or cough. Other important features of the disease are the extreme response of airways to various stimuli, with an elevated CD4+ in the airways, and specific chronic inflammation characterized by T helper type 2-Th2 lymphocytes and eosinophils. Genetic tendency, atopy and allergen exposure are important risk factors for asthma [14].

Morphological changes such as acute inflammation, inflammation shifting from acute to chronic state, and remodeling are observed and are associated with patients' clinical features [15]. Since allergic reaction and inflammation occur in the bronchial walls, pathological findings are also seen primarily in the bronchi and bronchiole walls [16].

2.1.2. Incidence and Epidemiology

Asthma is a common chronic disease affecting every age group. The distribution of the disease around the world varies from country to country and sometimes from one region to another within the country. Asthma is more prevalent (higher than 10%) in Australia, New Zealand, some Pacific islands while it is very rare (lower than 1%) in people from Southeast Asian countries, North American Indians and Eskimos [17]. The prevalence rate in Turkey is lower than those recorded in several western countries [18-20]. Asthma is very common in most of the industrialized countries with a frequency of 3-7%. In the United States (US), it is estimated that more than 26 million people are suffering from asthma [2].

In Turkey, the prevalence of asthma in primary school children ranged from 6% to 15% [21], while the adjusted prevalence among adults ranged from 4.0% to 4.8% (average 4.4%) [20].

The prevalence and severity of asthma have been increasing worldwide. In the US, the overall annual age-adjusted prevalence rate of self-reported asthma increased 42% between 1982 and 1992 and the age-adjusted mortality rate due to asthma increased by 40% from 1982 to 1991 [22].

Increased morbidity and mortality rates are more striking in smaller countries. In addition, the economic burden of asthma on society is also getting higher [23]. In the US alone, the total amount of direct and indirect expenditures associated with asthma exceeds $56 billion annually [5].

It is estimated that asthma affects about 300 million people worldwide. This figure is about 3.5 million people for Turkey [9].

2.1.3. Mortality and Morbidity

Asthma prevalence, morbidity, and severity show a gender difference that varies with age. In infancy, it is seen twice as often in boys than in girls, while in adolescence this rate is equal. The prevalence and morbidity of asthma in women over 20 years of age is higher than men [24].

Although mortality due to asthma is a rare entity, mortality rates have increased recently. According to the World Health Organization (WHO) data, around the world there are 250 000 deaths related to asthma every year [25]. Asthma morbidity is affected by various factors such as quality of life, health care, asthma severity, drug use, treatment costs, prevalence, and incidence [24].

2.1.4. Mechanisms of Asthma

Asthma is an inflammatory airway disease characterized by the activity of various inflammatory cells and many mediators, accompanied by physiopathological changes [26]. The inflammation in asthma is similar to the type of inflammation occurring during allergic diseases. This type of inflammation is characterized by an acute increase in activated mast cell and eosinophil counts, as well as increased levels of natural killer T-cells and helper Th2 lymphocytes [26]. It is known that more than a hundred different mediators play a role in asthma and mediate the complex inflammatory response in the airways. These mediators are chemokines, cysteinyl leukotrienes, cytokines, histamine, nitric oxide, and prostaglandin D2 [26].

Some patients have atopic asthma. Atopy is defined as the secretion of an excessive amount of immunoglobulin E (IgE) against environmental allergens. Various genetic and environmental factors play a role in the emergence of atopy [27]. Allergens, smoking, air pollution, and viral respiratory tract infections in childhood are the environmental factors that play a role in the development of asthma [26, 28]. These patients react to antigenic stimulation with specific IgE release from B-lymphocytes. The resulting reaction leads to the release of mediators, such as histamine and eosinophilic chemotactic factor, which are formed in mast cells, basophils and macrophages. This finally results in bronchoconstriction, increased mucus secretion and edema in the airways [29].

Inflammatory cell infiltration and edema, as well as structural changes in the airway wall, also play a role in the increase of wall thickness [30, 31]. Airway stenosis causes symptoms and physiological changes in asthma. Hypertrophy in airway smooth muscles, airway edema, airway wall thickening, and mucus hypersecretion are the factors contributing to airway stenosis [32, 33].

2.1.5. Pathogenesis

Asthma is a chronic disease characterized by airway inflammation, bronchial hyperreactivity and reversible airway obstruction. Bronchial mucosal biopsy examinations show inflammation and persistent structural changes of eosinophils, basophils, mast cells, and Th2 lymphocytes.

Almost all asthma patients have an increase in subepithelial connective tissue regardless of the duration of the disease and the degree of inflammation, and this is typical for asthma. However, structural changes such as epithelial desquamation, bronchial smooth muscle hypertrophy and hyperplasia and revascularization are also seen. Environmental stimuli, such as recurrent viral respiratory tract infections, exposure to allergens, internal and external irritants cause acute inflammatory attacks in the bronchial mucosa. Extremely responsive airways are easily contracted with various stimuli and symptoms occur.

In addition to the genetic predisposition for asthma, environmental factors also play very important roles. Many epidemiological studies in recent years show that there is a significant increase in the prevalence of asthma, especially in western countries. It is accepted that the increase in prevalence in short periods such as ten-to-twenty years cannot be explained by genetic factors and that changing environmental conditions are responsible for this increase. Decreased frequency of infectious diseases, vaccination, widespread use of antibiotics, cleaner and more hygienic environments are among the factors responsible for increased asthma prevalence in western countries. On the other hand asthma is less common in developing countries where oro-fecal contamination, infections, and endotoxins are more frequent. This view, which explains the role of environmental factors in asthma immune pathogenesis, is called the hygiene hypothesis [34].

In asthma, cytokines and growth factors released from chronic inflammatory cells such as eosinophils and lymphocytes lead to permanent changes in the bronchial subepithelial fibrosis, smooth muscle hypertrophy, revascularization and goblet cell hypertrophy, which are called remodeling [26]. A wide spectrum of mediators such as enzymes released from inflammatory cells, cytokines, prostaglandins, viral infections, and irritants cause a sustained stimulation of the bronchial mucosa and damage to the mucosa. All these findings suggest that asthma develops as a result of very complex genetic and environmental interactions.

2.1.6. Risk Factors

Asthma risk factors are classified as individual and environmental risk factors. The most important individual risk factor is a genetic predisposition. The prevalence of asthma is higher in children with a family (mother, father, sibling) history of asthma [35]. Similarly, in monozygotic twins who share the same environment, asthma is more common than dizygotic twins [36].

Atopy is the exaggerated IgE synthesis of an individual against an allergen. In epidemiological studies, it is shown that almost half of the asthma patients are atopic [37]. Atopy is an age-related risk factor for asthma. Atopy, especially in children under 3 years of age is considered as the most important risk factor for advanced asthma [38]. Bronchial hyperreactivity is a rapid and excessive contraction of bronchi. Asymptomatic bronchial hyperreactivity is considered as a risk factor for asthma [39].

Until adolescence, asthma is more common in boys. The reason is that boys are more likely to have narrow bronchial diameters at this age, higher airway resistance and slower airflow rates [40]. This risk is eliminated by the fact that changes in the rib cage with puberty only occur in men. In adolescence, the risk of asthma increases in girls.

One of the risk factors associated with the environment is the exposure of allergen-sensitive individuals to in-house and out-door allergens. However, it has not been determined whether exposure to an allergen is the cause of primary asthma or the occurrence and continuity of the complaints [41].

Upper respiratory tract infections in the early years of life reduce the risk of asthma in advanced age, while serious lower respiratory tract infections increase the risk. The prevalence of asthma in children with no siblings or only one sibling is higher than that of those with more than one sibling [42].

2.1.7. Diagnosis

Asthma is a clinical diagnosis. Diagnosis is often made with history, physical examination, laboratory tests, and treatment response [26].

2.1.7.1. Patient History

Recurrent chronic respiratory complaints play a key role in the diagnosis of asthma. Recurrent persistent dry cough and/or wheezing attacks, chest tightness and shortness of breath are the main symptoms of these complaints. Complaints increasing at night or awakening from sleep, triggered with common cold, physical activity, cold/dry air, irritants (cigarette smoke, odors, air pollution), inhaled allergens (such as pollen, house dust mites, mildew, cat, cockroach) are typical. The family (mother, father and sibling) history of asthma is also important for diagnosis. Previous good response to bronchodilator and corticosteroid treatment supports the diagnosis [26].

2.1.7.2. Physical Examination

- Upper respiratory tract (nasal secretion, mucosal swelling and/or nasal polyps)

- Chest (wheezing in normal breathing or long phase in exhalation, the width of the rib cage, use of auxiliary muscles, humped shoulder view, chest deformity) and,
- Skin (atopic dermatitis, eczema).

2.1.7.3. Spirometry

It is a recommended method to make an asthma diagnosis by measuring airflow restriction and reversibility. It enables clinicians to evaluate the reversibility and the obstruction in patients older than five years. Under most circumstances, short-acting beta2-agonist bronchodilators (salbutamol or terbutaline) are used to test reversibility. A positive diagnostic response to bronchodilators is an increase in FEV1 from the baseline that is more than 200 mL and more than 15% of the prebronchodilator value. Patients' perceptions of airway obstruction vary widely. Spirometry is a fundamental measure to diagnose asthma because medical history and physical examination are not reliable to assess pulmonary condition.

Commonly used pulmonary function test parameters are:

FVC (Forced vital capacity; L): It is the total amount of air excreted by a forced expiration after a maximum inspiration. It is over 80% in healthy individuals.

FEV1 (Forced expiratory volume in 1 second; L): It is the amount of air expelled in 1 second of forced expiration. It provides information about obstruction in large and middle-sized bronchi. Tests, where FEV1 is measured below one liter should not be evaluated as the sensitivity decreases. It is over 80% in healthy individuals. A 12% increase in FEV1 after bronchodilator administration compared to the initial value is expressed as reversibility and this supports the diagnosis of asthma [26].

FEV1/FVC (%): FEV1 can also be found to be low in other diseases apart from obstructive diseases. Therefore, it is more appropriate to consider the FEV1/FVC ratio. It is over 80% in healthy individuals.

FEF25-75 (Forced expiratory flow in 25-75% of FVC; L/min): It is the average flow rate between 25-75% of the forced vital capacity. It provides information about small- and middle-sized bronchi. It is over 70% in healthy individuals.

PEF (Peak expiratory flow; L/min): The peak expiratory flow rate in forced expiration after a maximum inspiration. The PEF value is measured in the morning before taking the medication and at night when the values are higher. The patient is monitored by PEF using a portable, inexpensive, simple tool called a peak flow meter. More than 20% variability between morning and evening PEF measurements, or 15% or more reversibility in the PEF after bronchodilator administration supports the diagnosis of asthma [26].

Spirometry is generally preferred to peak flow meter due to the wide variability of the peak flow meter measurements and the reference values. The peak flow meter is designed for monitoring; it is not a diagnostic tool [43].

Bronchial provocation tests: In patients with normal pulmonary function but having symptoms compatible with asthma, methacholine, histamine or exercise may be used to stimulate the bronchia. The test result is usually expressed as a dose (or concentration) provoking a 20% or more reduction in baseline at FEV1. This test is sensitive but not specific to asthma. This indicates that a negative test is useful for the exclusion of asthma in a patient who does not use inhaled corticosteroids. However, a positive test does not always mean that the patient has asthma [26, 45]; as airway sensitivity can also be found positive in diseases such as allergic rhinitis, cystic fibrosis, bronchiectasis or chronic obstructive pulmonary disease (COPD) [26].

Allergy tests: Atopy is the most important risk factor for asthma and supports the diagnosis in patients with suspected asthma. It is also important for environmental control. The assessment of atopy is determined by epidermal skin tests in vivo, by radioallergosorbent test (RAST) in vitro to detect specific IgE in circulating allergens. Skin tests are faster, simpler, cheaper and more sensitive than RAST [26].

2.1.8. Treatment

The first step of the treatment in asthma is to inform the patients and their families about the disease and to provide the physician-patient-pharmacist cooperation necessary for the treatment. The most important goal of asthma treatment is to provide full control in asthma.

According to the GINA 2018 Report, the aims of long-term asthma management are stated as follows:

- To prevent chronic and bothersome symptoms
- To carry on normal daily activities
- To provide normal pulmonary function
- To prevent asthma attacks
- To minimize adverse effects

In order to achieve these goals, asthma treatment should be applied and standardized within a certain program.

Treatment approaches are as follows:

- Patient education: Patients should be educated about the causes of asthma, chronic inflammation, drug properties, causes and symptoms of an attack, peak flow meter use, drug doses and, if necessary, increasing drug dosage. This should be continued at regular intervals.
- Abstain from triggering agents (in-house and out-door allergens, chemicals, infections, drugs, gastroesophageal reflux, etc.).
- Determination of the severity of the disease: The disease is graded by considering the severity and duration of symptoms and abnormalities of the pulmonary function tests.
- Medication treatment plan:
  Medications are categorized into three main groups: a) controller medications [inhaled corticosteroids (ICS), oral corticosteroids, leukotriene receptor antagonists (LTRA), long-acting beta2-agonists (LABA), and theophylline)] b) reliever (rescue)

medications [short-acting beta2-agonists (SABA), theophylline, and inhaled anticholinergic agents] c) Add-on therapies for patients with severe asthma (high dose ICS and LABA).

Table 1. Classification of asthma severity (≥ 12 years of age)

Intermittent
• Symptoms < 2 days/week
• Nighttime awakenings ≤ 2/month
• Short-acting beta2-agonist use for symptom control (not for the prevention of exercise-induced bronchoconstriction) ≤ 2 days/week
• No activity limitation
• Pulmonary function test FEV1 > 80% predicted
• FEV1/FVC normal*
• Normal FEV1 between exacerbations
• FEV1 or PEF variability < 20%
Mild Persistent
• Symptoms > 2 days/week but not daily
• Nighttime awakenings 3-4/month
• Short-acting beta2-agonist use for symptom control (not for the prevention of exercise-induced bronchoconstriction) > 2 days/week but not daily and ≤ 1/day
• Minor activity limitation
• Pulmonary function test FEV1 ≥ 80% predicted
• FEV1/FVC normal
• FEV1 or PEF variability < 20-30%
Moderate Persistent
• Symptoms daily
• Nighttime awakenings > 1/week but not nightly
• Short-acting beta2-agonist use for symptom control (not for the prevention of exercise-induced bronchoconstriction) daily
• Some activity limitation
• Pulmonary function test FEV1 60-80% predicted
• FEV1/FVC decreased 5%
• FEV1 or PEF variability > 30%
Severe Persistent
• Symptoms throughout the day
• Nighttime awakenings often 7/week
• Short-acting beta2-agonist use for symptom control (not for the prevention of exercise-induced bronchoconstriction) several times per day
• Extremely activity limitation
• Pulmonary function test FEV1 < 60% predicted
• FEV1/FVC decreased > 5%
• FEV1 or PEF variability > 30%

*Normal FEV1/FVC: 8-19 years 85%, 20-39 years 80%, 40-59 years 75%, 60-80 years 70%.

Four categories of asthma severity are summarized in Table 1 [46]. The severity of asthma can change from patient to patient and from time to time in the same patient; the basic rule of treatment is to adjust the dose and type of the medication according to the severity. The method of adjusting the treatment according to the severity of asthma is called stepwise treatment. The medication treatment used according to the severity of asthma is presented in Table 2.

Asthma treatment steps can be listed as follows:

1) Determination of asthma control level
2) Adjustment of treatment to control asthma
3) Monitoring the asthma control status

Table 2. Medication treatment according to the severity of asthma

Severity	Controller Medications	Alternative Treatments
Intermittent	Not necessary	-
Mild Persistent	Inhaled corticosteroids (ICS) (100-400 µg budesonide or equivalent)	• Theophylline • Cromolyn • Leukotriene antagonist
Moderate Persistent	ICS (400-800 µg budesonide or equivalent)	• ICS + theophylline • ICS + long-acting bronchodilator • Higher dose ICS • ICS + leukotriene antagonist
Severe Persistent	ICS (800 µg budesonide or equivalent) + one or more of the following treatments • Extended-release theophylline • Long-acting β2-agonist • Leukotriene antagonist • Oral corticosteroid	-

2.1.9. Determination of Asthma Control Level

The asthma control levels of patients should be evaluated both before and after treatment.

2.1.9.1. Criteria Used in the Estimation of Asthma Control

- Asthma signs and symptoms

- Asthma control questionnaires
- Pulmonary function
  - Pulmonary function tests
  - Monitoring the peak flow rates
- Asthma exacerbation history
- Medications and adverse effects
- Communication between patient and family; and patient satisfaction
- Minimally invasive markers
  - Airway hypersensitivity
  - Eosinophilia in sputum or blood
  - Exhaled nitric oxide (FENO)
  - Pharmacogenetics of asthma treatment

2.1.9.2. Symptoms Assessed in the Estimation of Asthma Control

Presence of the following 4 symptoms is questioned:

- Daytime asthma symptoms (wheezing, cough, tightness of chest or shortness of breath)
- Nighttime awakenings
- Frequency of short-acting beta2-agonist use
- Activity limitation (including exercise)

In international guidelines, several tests have been developed to determine asthma control status in a short time. These tests, validated for evaluating clinical control in asthma, provide numerical values to distinguish between different levels of asthma control. These tests include various parameters such as the clinical parameters (symptom scores, daytime shortness of breath, nighttime awakenings, bronchodilator requirement), pulmonary function tests (PEF and FEV1), subjective parameters of asthma control and bronchial hypersensitivity, eosinophilia in induced sputum and the level of FENO.

The most commonly used tests are:

1) Asthma Control Questionnaire (ACQ)
2) Asthma Therapy Assessment Questionnaire (ATAQ)
3) Asthma Control Test (ACT)
4) Asthma Impact Survey (AIS-6)
5) Asthma Control Scoring System (ACSS)

Asthma Therapy Assessment Questionnaire (ATAQ): It is useful in assessing the risk in young adult asthma patients without a previous history of acute attack. A high score indicates a control problem [47].

Asthma Control Questionnaire (ACQ): This questionnaire was developed by Juniper et al. [48]. It consists of six questions and an additional FEV1 value.

Each question is given a score between 0 and 6. In the seventh question, the FEV1 value was scored between 0 and 6 (0: >95%predicted, 6: <50% predicted). The questionnaire score is the average of 7 questions and the mean score is interpreted as '≤0.75: fully controlled, 0.75-1.5: partly controlled, ≥1.5: not controlled [9, 48]'. Stable and uncontrolled asthma groups have shown that ACQ can significantly differentiate changes (improvement or impairment) in the clinical status. A significant correlation was found between ACQ and AQLQ, Medical Outcomes Survey Short Form-36 (SF-36), and the evaluations of clinicians [49].

Asthma Control Scoring System (ACSS): ACSS consists of respiratory symptoms, FEV1 and eosinophilia percent in sputum [50].

Asthma Control Test (ACT™): It was developed as a simple method that can be used by patients and physicians to detect uncontrolled patients while assessing asthma control. It is a questionnaire consisting of five questions taking into consideration the criteria such as asthma symptoms, the use of reliever medication and the effect of asthma on daily life. In addition, it allows the evaluation of asthma control in patients with unrated FEV1.

It is simpler than ACQ and is reported to be more comprehensive than ATAQ in determining the level of asthma control [51]. The reliability and validity of ACT were demonstrated in asthma patients who have not been previously evaluated by a specialist [51-54].

The maximum score is 25 and the minimum score is 5. A score of 20-25 indicates that the disease is well controlled; a score of 16-19 indicates that it is partly controlled and a score of 5-15 indicates that it is uncontrolled [26].

Recent studies have reported that pulmonary function tests and ACT have similar results in determining uncontrolled patients [53].

According to the classification approach based on the level of asthma control, asthma is classified as 'well controlled, partly controlled and uncontrolled'.

Global Initiative for Asthma (GINA) diagnosis and treatment guidelines may also be used to define asthma control status [26] (Table 3).

2.1.9.3. Control-Based Asthma Management

According to the GINA guidelines, the current treatment approach focuses on asthma control. The treatment approach is arranged in five steps, where the treatment intensity (dose and/or the number of drugs) can be increased to provide control. A symptom-relieving drug should be given at all steps as needed. From step 2 to step 5, a variety of controlling drugs are used. If control is not achieved with the current treatment, treatment is gradually increased until control is achieved. If control is maintained for at least 3 months, treatment may be gradually decreased until the lowest treatment step and treatment dose is reached (Table 4).

Table 3. Levels of asthma control

Asthma Symptoms	Well controlled	Partly controlled	Uncontrolled
In the past 4 weeks, has the patient had: - Daytime asthma symptoms ≥2/week - Activity limitation - Nighttime awakenings - Reliever needed for symptoms ≥2/week	None of these	1-2 of these	3-4 of these
Asthma Control Test scores	20-25	16-19	5-15

2.1.10. Medications Used in Asthma Treatment

The medications used for asthma management are classified into two groups as controller and reliever medications (Table 5). Controller medications provide long-term control. These are inhaled and systemic steroids, cromolyn sodium (sodium cromoglycate), nedocromil sodium, leukotriene antagonists, long-acting theophylline, and long-acting beta2-agonists. Reliever medications are used to treat bronchospasm and bronchial obstruction and supposed to be used when needed. These are short-acting beta2-agonists, theophylline (i.v. form) and anticholinergics [9].

Asthma medications can be administered through inhalation, oral or parenteral routes. The main advantage of inhaled therapy is reduced systemic adverse effects and the direct delivery of medications to the airways, resulting in high local concentrations. Increased use of reliever medication indicates a worsening of asthma control. This requires the re-evaluation of treatment. The aim of asthma treatment is to maintain clinical control.

2.1.10.1. Glucocorticoids

Steroids are the most effective anti-inflammatory drugs for asthma control. Oral or intravenous steroids are life-saving in the asthma attack; however, they are not for long-term use due to their adverse effects. Thus, inhaled steroids are used for long-term asthma control. Studies indicate that inhaled corticosteroids reduce asthma symptoms as well as frequency and severity of exacerbations, improve quality of life, increase pulmonary function, and decrease asthma-related mortality [55, 56]. They are used in increasing doses depending on the severity of asthma. If at least one of the relevant criteria mentioned in Table 3 is present for a particular patient, then the patient should be prescribed a high dose of inhaled steroid. After adequate control, each dose is reduced by 25% every 1-3 month to reach the lowest effective dose [9].

Inhaled corticosteroids provide the greatest benefit at low doses (400 µg budesonide per day or equivalent) (Table 6). The use of higher doses provides a small amount of additional benefit in terms of asthma control while increasing the risk of adverse effects. Smoking reduces the response to inhaled corticosteroids, thus smokers may require higher doses.

Table 4. The stepwise approach to control symptoms in adults, adolescents, and children 6-11 years (GINA guideline 2018) [26]

⟨ DECREASE   **Treatment Steps**   INCREASE ⟩

	STEP 1	STEP 2	STEP 3	STEP 4	STEP 5
Preferred controller of choice		Low dose ICS	Low dose ICS/LABA[a]	Med/high ICS/LABA	Refer for add-on treatment e.g., tiotropium[b,c], anti-IgE, anti-IL5[b]
Other controller options	Consider low dose ICS	LTRA Low dose theoph[b]	Med/high dose ICS Low dose ICS + LTRA (or + theoph[b])	Add tiotropium[b,c] Med/high dose ICS + LTRA (or + theoph[b])	Add low dose OCS
Reliever	As-needed SABA			As-needed SABA or low dose ICS/formoterol[d]	

ICS: inhaled corticosteroid; LABA: long-acting β2 agonist; LTRA: leukotriene receptor antagonist; med: medium; OCS: oral corticosteroid; SABA: short-acting β2 agonist; theoph: theophylline; [a]For children 6-11 years, the preferred Step 3 treatment is medium dose ICS; [b]Not for children <12 years; [c]Tiotropium by mist inhaler is an add-on treatment for patients with a history of exacerbations; it is not indicated in children <12 years; [d]Low dose ICS/formoterol is the reliever medication for patients prescribed low dose budesonide/formoterol or low dose beclomethasone/formoterol maintenance and reliever therapy.

In order to provide clinical control, it may be preferable to add a second controller medication to the inhaled glucocorticosteroid instead of increasing the steroid dose [57-59].

In the treatment of chronic asthma systemic steroids are added to the treatment if adequate control cannot be achieved by the combined use of high-dose inhaled steroids and long-acting bronchodilators. They can be used for short periods or longer periods if necessary. They can also be used orally or intravenously in the treatment of attacks [9].

Oral corticosteroids cause many adverse reactions such as osteoporosis, peripheral myopathy, and cataract. Inhaled corticosteroids are known to cause topical adverse effects such as oropharyngeal candidiasis and hoarseness due to pharyngeal accumulation [60].

Table 5. Medications used for asthma management

Controller Medications	Reliever Medications
1- Inhaled steroids	1- Short-acting β2-agonists
• Budesonide	• Terbutaline
• Fluticasone	• Salbutamol
• Beclomethasone	2- Theophylline
2- Leukotriene receptor antagonists	3- Anticholinergics
• Montelukast	• Ipratropium bromide
• Zafirlukast	
3- Long-acting β2-agonists	
• Formoterol	
• Salmeterol	
4- Extended-release theophylline	

Table 6. Daily equivalent doses of inhaled steroids in adults

Inhaled steroids	Low dose (µg)	Medium dose (µg)	High dose (µg)
Beclomethasone dipropionate (CFC)	250-500	500-1000	1000-2000
Beclomethasone dipropionate (HFA)	100-200	200-400	400-800
Budesonide*	200-400	400-800	800-1600
Fluticasone	100-250	250-500	500-1000
Ciclesonide*	80-160	160-320	320-1280

*A single dose can be used daily; CFC: chloro fluoro carbon; HFA: hydrofluoro alkane.

2.1.10.2. Leukotriene Modifying Medications

As a result of allergen exposure, leukotrienes and histamine are secreted together with many mediators in the nasal mucosa. Leukotrienes and histamine are both early and late phase mediators of allergic rhinitis.

Histamine is one of the mediators that cause nasal itching, rhinorrhea and sneezing, while leukotrienes cause nasal congestion, and rhinorrhea. In many studies, it was observed that there is a correlation between leukotrienes and rhinitis symptoms after exposure to nasal allergens [61].

Leukotrienes (LTC_4), (LTD_4), (LTE_4) are a group of arachidonic acid-derived endogenous substances synthesized via the 5-lipoxygenase pathway. Leukotrienes are powerful inflammatory eicosanoids released from various cells including mast cells, basophils, and eosinophils. They are also components of the slow-reacting agent of anaphylaxis.

They bind to cysteinyl leukotriene receptors in human airways and cause a number of airway activities such as mucus secretion, enhancing vascular permeability, bronchoconstriction, and eosinophil accumulation.

Leukotriene synthesis inhibitor (zileuton) and receptor antagonists (zafirlukast, montelukast, pranlukast, pobilukast, tomelukast, verlukast) are used to eliminate these effects.

Clinical studies have shown that these drugs have a small and variable bronchodilator effect, reduce symptoms including cough [62], improve pulmonary function, and reduce airway inflammation and asthma exacerbations. However, when used alone as a controller, their effects are less than those of the low-dose inhaled glucocorticosteroids; therefore, they cannot replace these medications. Leukotriene modifying medications may reduce the dose of inhaled glucocorticosteroids in moderate and severe asthma when used as add-on therapy; they may improve asthma control. In terms of prevention of exacerbations, they were reported to be less effective than long-acting β2-agonists as add-on therapy.

2.1.10.3. Leukotriene Receptor Antagonists

Leukotriene receptor antagonists had been developed in the treatment of asthma for many years and entered the market in the 90s [63].

2.1.10.4. Zafirlukast

Zafirlukast is available in 20 mg and 10 mg oral tablets. Zafirlukast is the competitive antagonist of LTC_4, LTD_4, LTE_4 receptors and it is a highly selective and potent peptide. The maximum level in plasma is reached after 3 hours and the half-life is about 10 hours. Approximately 99% of zafirlukast binds to plasma proteins and especially to albumin. It is metabolized in the liver and excreted in the feces. It is used as 20 mg twice daily. Food reduces its bioavailability by 40%; therefore it is recommended to be taken 1 hour before or 2 hours after meals. It should not be used in children under 12 years. It is indicated for allergic rhinitis, asthma, and bronchospasm prophylaxis.

It is contraindicated in cases of liver failure or cirrhosis. Although it may cause a slight increase in serum transaminases, this increase is temporary and asymptomatic. Some systemic eosinophilia cases, including Churg-Strauss syndrome, were reported; however, a correlation was not found. Studies with oral anticoagulants suggested no recommendations except for monitoring of prothrombin time. It should not be used in pregnant women and nursing mothers.

There is no interaction with other respiratory system medications. It can be used with other treatments administered in the treatment of asthma and allergy.

2.1.10.5. Montelukast

There are 10 mg film tablets (adult), 5 or 4 mg chewable tablet (child) formulations on the market. Montelukast strongly inhibits the physiological effects of LTC_4, LTD_4, and LTE_4 in cysteinyl leukotriene CysLT1 receptor without showing any agonist activity.

It reaches the peak plasma concentration within 3 hours on an empty stomach; the bioavailability is 66% for the tablet and 73% for the chewable tablet. Approximately 99% is bound to plasma proteins. Oral absorption is not significantly affected by food. All medications and metabolites are excreted via the bile.

It is indicated for prophylactic and chronic treatment of asthma and allergic rhinitis. It should not be used in pregnant women and nursing mothers.

There is no significant pharmacokinetic interaction with theophylline, corticosteroids, oral contraceptives and oral anticoagulants. No dose adjustment is required in mild to moderate liver failure and renal failure.

The recommended dose for asthma maintenance therapy is 4 mg daily in the evening, in children 12 months to 5 years; 5 mg daily in the evening, in children 6 to 14 years, and 10 mg daily in the evening in patients 15 years and older.

2.1.10.6. Beta-2 Agonists

β2 agonists are used to treat asthma due to the following effects:

- They provide bronchodilation.
- They increase mucus secretion and mucociliary clearance.
- They reduce microvascular permeability by epithelial ion and water transport.
- They inhibit sympathetic and parasympathetic transmission.
- They prevent the mediator release from the mast cells and other inflammatory cells.
- They are protective against exercise, cold, dry air and allergens.

Beta2-agonists can be classified according to their durations of action and peak plasma time as presented in Table 7.

Table 7. Classification of beta2-agonists according to durations of action and peak plasma time

Fast-, short-acting	Fast-, medium-acting	Long-acting
• Epinephrine • Norepinephrine • Dopamine • Isoproterenol (β1-β2)	• Terbutaline • Salbutamol • Fenoterol • Pirbuterol • Bitolterol • Metaproterenol	• Formoterol (fast) • Salmeterol (slow)

Table 8. Comparison of long-acting beta2-agonists

Formoterol	Salmeterol
• β2/β1 selectivity is 400/1 • The effect on the bronchial smooth muscle is 86% • Bronchodilator effect starts in 3 minutes, lasts longer than 12 hours (stored in plasma)	• β2/β1 selectivity is 85000/1 • The effect on the bronchial smooth muscle is 62% • Bronchodilator effect starts in 10-11 minutes, lasts longer than 12 hours

Short- and medium-acting beta2-agonists are recommended to be used as a reliever in all stages of asthma as needed [26], while long-acting beta2-agonists (Table 8) are used in addition to the steroids in order to control symptoms more quickly. The adverse effects of beta2-agonists include tremor (most common), reflex tachycardia, hypokalemia, and hyperglycemia.

2.1.10.7. Methylxanthines

Xanthine group drugs (theophylline and aminophylline) are nonselective phosphodiesterase inhibitors that act by increasing intracellular cyclic adenosine monophosphate (c-AMP) levels in airway smooth muscles; they act as bronchodilators and smooth muscle relaxants, which relax the smooth muscles in bronchi and pulmonary blood vessels [64, 65].

Xanthine toxicity is dose-dependent. The bronchodilator effect of xanthine is best observed when given in doses close to toxic doses; this is a risk factor for toxicity and leads to difficulties in clinical use [60].

Although the narrow therapeutic range of xanthine derivatives leads to difficulties in clinical use, extended-release preparations used in recent years eliminate this condition and provide a constant serum concentration by the administration of 1 or 2 doses per day.

During theophylline use, blood levels should be regularly measured, dose and product changes should be considered, and patients should continue treatment at the lowest effective dose (recommended blood level is 8-14 μg/mL) [66, 67]. Adverse reactions due to increased theophylline blood levels are as presented in Table 9.

Table 9. Adverse reactions due to increased theophylline blood levels [67]

Theophylline Serum Level (μg/mL)	Adverse Reactions
15-25	Abdominal pain, nausea, vomiting, diarrhea, muscle cramp, headache, agitation
25-35	Tachycardia, arrhythmia, convulsion
> 35	Ventricular tachycardia, ataxia

Theophylline is the most commonly used xanthine derivative, metabolized by cytochrome P450. The clearance of the drug decreases with age. Many other physiological parameters and medications change theophylline metabolism [60].

2.1.10.8. Chromones

Sodium cromoglycate and nedocromil sodium are effective agents for the treatment of long-term asthma. Their anti-inflammatory effects are poor and they are less effective than low dose inhaled glucocorticosteroid therapy. A minimum period of 2 weeks is required for response to treatment. Maximum effect can be observed after 4-6 weeks. If improvement is not achieved at this period, inhaled steroids are indicated. They prevent symptoms during long-term use, prevent asthma attacks if used shortly before exercise or known allergen exposure, and prevent bronchospasms caused by inhalation of cold, dry air and sulfur dioxide. There are no significant adverse effects [9].

2.1.10.9. Anti-IgE

The use of anti-IgE (e.g., omalizumab) is a treatment option limited to patients with high serum IgE levels. Omalizumab is currently indicated in patients with severe allergic asthma that cannot be controlled by inhaled glucocorticosteroid therapy. It reduces symptoms, reliever medication use and exacerbations.

Omalizumab is a recombinant DNA derivative human monoclonal antibody that selectively binds to immunoglobulin E (IgE) in humans.

Omalizumab binds IgE and reduces the amount of free IgE that will trigger a sequence of allergic events by inhibiting the binding of this immunoglobulin to high-affinity IgE receptors (FceR1).

2.1.10.10. Anticholinergics (Ipratropium Bromide)

Anticholinergics are used alternatively in the treatment of severe bronchospasm and severe chronic asthma in addition to beta2-agonists or in the patient group where beta2-agonists cannot be used due to adverse effects. It is the medication of choice for the treatment of asthma attacks caused by beta-blockers. Tachycardia and arrhythmia effects are less frequent than those observed with beta-agonists [9].

2.1.10.11. Routes of Medication Administration

Medications used in the treatment of asthma may be given to patients through different routes (inhaler, oral, parenteral). In the asthma treatment, inhalation is the preferred route due to the fact that medication can be given directly to the airways, their effects start in a short time, and systemic adverse effects are minimal. For this purpose spray dosage forms such as metered dose inhalers can be used. The appropriate use of inhalation medications, thus optimum treatment outcomes depend on patient compliance. Therefore, asthma patients who are prescribed inhaled medications should receive patient education on inhalation techniques and it should be checked at every visit whether they are using their inhalers correctly [9].

Another form of inhalers is the dry powder inhaler. Their inhaler technique is slightly different and easier than that of metered-dose inhalers. The patient inhales the powder medication with a fast and deep inspiration; therefore dry powder inhalers may not be effective in patients with very low inspiratory flow rates. The dry powder can be moistened if the patient accidentally breathes into the inhaler.

Nebulizers are electrical devices, which deliver the medication to the patient by inhalation; they decompose the medication into small particles by the use of high pressure or ultrasound. When the metered-dose inhalers are used with a spacer device by appropriate technic and at adequate doses, they are as effective as the nebulizers. Nebulizers may be preferred in elderly patients who cannot adapt, in infants and at severe attacks. They should be available at the service and emergency department at any time. Asthma medications should be given in children under two years of age with a nebulizer or spacer with a facial mask. Children can learn to use sprays with spacer from the age of three. Dry powder inhalers can be used in children over seven years old [9].

2.1.11. Preventive Treatment

The first step of prevention is improving the home environment. Elimination of factors that cause house dust will reduce or prevent the symptoms of home dust allergies. Mites found mainly in beds, carpets, cushions, and furniture should be eliminated. Foods that have been identified as allergic should not be consumed [68].

2.1.11.1. Reduction of Exposure to Risk Factors in Asthma

Important allergens are aeroallergens or inhaled allergens. The inhalation of the antigenic particles in the air through the respiratory tract causes a reaction [69].

Information is given below about the most common allergens.

House dust mites
- Ventilation should be increased; moisture should be prevented.
- Leather, artificial leather, wood and plastic goods should be preferred.
- Masks can be used when doing housework.
- Cleaning with wet cloth should be done after sweeping.
- At least one cleaning per week should be done with a strong vacuum cleaner.
- Humidifier devices should not be used.
- Feathered and stuffed toys should not be kept at home.
- Bed linen should be washed at least at 55 °C once a week.
- Synthetic pillows must be used instead of wool, cotton or feather pillows.
- Removable carpets should be removed.

Grass and tree pollen
- Individuals should not go out during the pollen-spreading period of the specific plants, which cause sensitivity.
- During the pollen propagation period of the specific plants, doors and windows should be kept closed.

- Pollen filters should be used at home and in the car.
- Mask and eyeglasses must be worn; contact lenses should not be used.
- When coming home from outside, a shower should be taken and the outdoor clothes should be changed.

Smoking and in-door air pollution
- Smoking makes people more prone to asthma development (especially in childhood exposure). Active and second-hand smoking should be strictly avoided.
- Formaldehyde from stoves, furnace fuels, fried oils, air fresheners, paint and polishing, CO, CO_2, NO_2, SO_2 must be avoided by providing good ventilation.
- Cleaning should not be done with irritant substances.

2.1.12. Measurement of Airflow Limitation (Spirometry)

In order to detect patients in the early stages of the disease, spirometry should be performed in all patients with chronic cough and sputum, and a history of risk factor exposure, even if there is no dyspnea. Pulmonary function tests are the most commonly used parameters for the diagnosis of asthma and the determination of the etiology as well as for the assessment of disease severity, response to treatment and prognosis.

Spirometry should measure the maximal air volume excreted by forced expiration from the maximum inspiration point (forced vital capacity, FVC), and the volume of air expelled in the first second of this maneuver (forced expiratory volume in the 1st second, FEV1) and the ratio of these two measurements (FEV1/FVC) should be calculated. In patients with asthma, both FEV1 and FVC are typically low. The postbronchodilator FEV1 <80% (predicted) with FEV1/FVC <70% indicates the presence of a non-reversible airflow limitation. The FEV1/FVC ratio is sensitive enough to measure airflow limitation and FEV1/FVC <70% is considered to be an early indicator of airflow limitation in patients with FEV1 >80% predicted within normal limits (FEV1).

2.2. Quality of Life

While the importance of quality of life is emphasized at various literature, a universally accepted definition does not exist [70, 71].

The World Health Organization defines the quality of life as the perception of life in relation to its goals, expectations, standards, and interests within the framework of culture and value systems. It is a broad concept that is influenced in a complex way from the person's physical health, psychological state, beliefs, social relations and the relationship with the environment. This definition reflects the fact that quality of life is a subjective assessment that is deeply embedded in cultural, social and environmental concepts [72].

2.2.1. Health-Related Quality of Life

Health-related quality of life is a multidimensional term that includes the disease-affected aspect of quality of life [71]. Health-related quality of life shows how 'good' the individual feels for himself/herself in terms of occupational, emotional, social and physical dimensions; and their feelings about how a particular disease affects the functionality of the individual in these dimensions [73].

The physical dimension is related to a person's perception of how much he/she can fulfill his/her daily work by using energy. The social dimension includes the degree to which a person can relate to and interact with individuals such as family members, neighbors, colleagues, and others. The psychological dimension consists of emotional and mental conditions such as depression, anxiety, fear, anger, and happiness [70].

Health-related quality of life scales were developed in order to investigate the disease process and treatment in the daily life of the patient, to determine the effectiveness of the treatment from the patient's perspective and to determine the patient's social, emotional and physical needs throughout the disease. These scales are used to decide between different treatments, to inform the patient about the efficacy of the treatment, to monitor the success of the treatment from the patient's perspective [74].

2.2.2. Scales Used in Health-Related Quality of Life Measurement

The scales used in the assessment of health-related quality of life are classified into two groups as 'general-purpose (generic) scales' and 'special-purpose (specific) scales'.

General-purpose scales are scales used in the general population, which can be applied to various health conditions and diseases. They may be less sensitive to disease-specific conditions due to not being designed for a specific disease and may not detect small changes in quality of life [75]. Short Form-36, Nottingham Health Profile, Euro-QOL, Wellness Scale, Disease Impact Profile and World Health Organization Quality of Life Questionnaire are frequently used health-related quality of life scales.

Special-purpose scales are specific to a specific population (children, seniors, adolescents), specific status (pain), specific disease (diabetes, epilepsy, rheumatoid arthritis) or a specific function. The main advantage of the special-purpose scales is that they can measure the change related to the medical intervention more sensitively; the disadvantages are that they cannot handle the person as a whole and cannot compare between different situations and programs [73]. Saint George's Respiratory Questionnaire (SGRQ), Arthritis Impact Measurement Scale (AIMS), Asthma Quality of Life Questionnaire (AQLQ), Diabetes Quality of Life (DQOL), Kidney Disease Quality of Life (KDQOL), Quality of Life in Epilepsy (QOLIE), HIV Overview of Problems-Evaluation System (HOPES) can be given as examples of special-purpose scales [75].

Quality of life questionnaires also have some disadvantages. Although there are shortened versions, it generally takes 10 minutes to administer. The questionnaires measure the patient's current functional recovery and do not provide information about how asthma will affect the patient's future life [54]. For example, even if a specific treatment improves the current quality of life of a patient, it can hardly treat the inflammatory damage that could lead to future damage; but an optimistic patient may still appear to have a high quality of life. Therefore, quality of life measures should be supported by clinical parameters such as FEV1 or PEF measurements, which are more objective parameters of asthma control [54, 76].

2.2.3. Quality of Life in Asthma

As a chronic condition, asthma affects the patient's physical, psychological and social health as well as the quality of life. Measuring the quality of life in patients with chronic respiratory diseases allows better understanding of the benefits of a treatment [44, 77, 78].

Despite optimal pharmacological treatment, the most important problems in asthma patients are respiratory distress and activity restriction. When FEV1 falls below one liter, shortness of breath causes significant deterioration of a patient's daily life and activities. In advanced disease, emotional and social functions, self-care, mobility, and sleep are severely affected [79].

Quality of life questionnaires allow measuring the extent to which the disease affects the patient's daily life as well as his health and happiness. Both generic and disease-specific quality of life questionnaires are used in patients with asthma.

Quality of life information, as one of the most important health outcomes, has been widely used in the evaluation of medicines in clinical trials. The clinical applications of quality of life analysis can be listed as follows [80]:

- Identification of unexpected health problems
- Monitoring the course of the disease or response to treatment
- Increasing the communication between the healthcare provider and the patient

2.2.4. Asthma Quality of Life Questionnaire (AQLQ)

Asthma Quality of Life Questionnaire (AQOL) is a disease-specific questionnaire consisting of 32 questions, validated for the measurement of functional impairment in adults with asthma. Responses are evaluated with a 7-point Likert scale (1: severely impaired, 7: not impaired at all). It measures functional impairment during the last two weeks. AQLQ consists of 4 domains; namely 'symptoms (11 items), activity limitation (12 items, 5 of which are individualized), emotional function (5 items) and environmental exposure (4 items)'. Mean scores are calculated for the total questionnaire and for each domain [81, 82].

The domains of the questionnaire are as follows [82]:

- Asthma symptoms: shortness of breath, chest tightness, wheezing, feeling of heaviness in the chest, cough, morning symptoms, nighttime awakenings
- Activity limitation: avoidance or restriction of activities due to asthma
- Environmental exposure: cigarette smoke, dust, air pollution, strong odors
- Emotional function: worrying about asthma, disappointment, worrying about taking medications, being afraid of not having the medications with them, being afraid of not breathing

This scale developed by Juniper et al. [82] was shown to be a valid questionnaire for the evaluation of the quality of life in asthma patients and was reported to be sensitive to detecting changes in quality of life in asthma.

2.3. Pharmacist's Role in Asthma Management

Patients with chronic diseases often require more complex treatment regimens. Therefore, the patient's adherence may be low, medication-induced adverse effects may be observed, hospitalization rates, health expenses, and morbidity and mortality rates may increase. Medication-related events may require the pharmacist's professional approach [75].

The pharmacist has an important role in the ongoing asthma treatment and in assisting patients throughout this process. There are many important areas where the pharmacist is active in improving the care of asthma patients.

Before receiving a diagnosis of asthma, many patients experience the effects of the disease in their daily activities. Pharmacists recognizing these symptoms may refer the patient to a respiratory disease specialist. The pharmacist has an important role in identification of the patients with asthma symptoms who visit the pharmacy or those who regularly buy OTC cough medications and those with recurrent antibiotic prescriptions. Early diagnosis of these patients may lead to timely medical treatment and non-pharmacologic measures such as smoking cessation and exercise.

Patient education alone cannot improve exercise performance or pulmonary function, but may play a role in improving skills to cope with the illness, and improving health status. The patient's inadequate knowledge of his/her condition may affect the treatment negatively and this may result in a lower quality of life. In accordance with the patient's consent, patients, their caregiver or family should also be clearly educated about asthma. Many pharmacists know about the family history and social status of their patients, and they should use this information to provide personalized care and education about the disease.

Another role of the pharmacists is helping to prevent asthma through health promotion activities. The role of the pharmacist in health promotion is not new and pharmacists have been active in this field for many years. Smoking cessation is the most important factor in preventing the decline of pulmonary function and is effective in all asthma treatment steps. The advice given by the healthcare professionals to quit smoking is a strong, motivating factor. The pharmacists are the most frequently encountered health care professionals and at an ideal position to consult those who want to quit smoking. They also play a key role in the provision of OTC products such as nicotine replacement therapies. They should also encourage asthma patients to receive their yearly influenza vaccines.

Patients should be educated on inhalation techniques, the triggering factors and ways to avoid them, how to monitor the disease status with the peak flow meter, identification of asthma symptoms, and how to seek appropriate medical help [83, 84].

Medication treatment in asthma is not curative. If the treatment does not have a positive effect on the patient's symptoms or exercise tolerance, the patient should consult his/her physician for re-evaluation. The pharmacist can review the patients' medication treatment and resolve medication-related problems such as non-compliance, wrong inhalation technique, and adverse effects; therefore, they can help prevent asthma crises and unnecessary hospitalizations. The pharmacist should confirm whether the patients are receiving appropriate pharmacological treatment for their asthma severity levels and that their medications are regularly reviewed by the physician.

Choice of the inhalation device should be personalized by considering the acceptability of the patient and the practical effectiveness of the device. While many patients cannot effectively coordinate their breath with the metered-dose inhaler, they can use a nebulizer, dry powder inhalers or spacer. The pharmacist must ensure that the patient is using the inhaler correctly. Patients often need someone to demonstrate the inhaler technique. Pharmacists should always provide this assistance to patients who come to the pharmacy to buy an inhaler.

The key roles undertaken by the pharmacist in the pharmaceutical care of the asthma patient are early identification of asthma patients, reduction of risk factors for asthma development such as smoking, and monitoring of the treatment. Pharmacists' understanding of the changes in asthma control status will enable them to be more actively involved in the patient identification process, selection of the inhalation device, teaching the inhaler technique and in the long-term monitoring of pulmonary function.

3. METHODS

This observational study [protocol no. PMS-208] was approved by the Ministry of Health of Turkey, General Directorate of Pharmaceuticals and Pharmacy with the decision No. B-10-0-IEG-0-15-00-01, dated 26.03.2010.

3.1. Subjects

All asthma patients admitted to the outpatient clinics of the Yedikule Training and Research Hospital for Chest Diseases and Thoracic Surgery for their follow-up controls, during the study period and met the inclusion criteria were informed about the study; those who accepted to participate and gave their informed consent were included in the study (n=50).

Inclusion criteria were being >18 and <65 years of age, and being prescribed a leukotriene receptor antagonist at the visit that happened on the day of the admittance. Those who used or have been using leukotriene receptor antagonists before this study, as well as the pregnant and lactating women were excluded from the study.

3.2. Data Collection

The first day of the hospital admittance of the patients who accepted to participate in the study, when, a leukotriene receptor antagonist was prescribed as add-on therapy to their current therapies, was recorded as the 'initial visit'. At the initial visit, the demographic and clinical features of the patients, as well as their medication-related information, were collected using standard data collection sheets. The asthma-related clinical status of the patients as represented by the FEV1%, FVC%, and FEV1/FVC values was recorded. On the other hand, asthma control status of the patients was determined according to the criteria of the GINA guidelines [84] as well as by using the Turkish versions of the Asthma Control Test [ACT]. The asthma-related quality of life of the patients was assessed by the Turkish version of the Asthma Quality of Life Questionnaire [AQLQ]. The scores obtained at the first visit were recorded as 'initial scores'.

At the initial visit, patients were prescribed montelukast and they were told to use this medication for three months. The 'control visits' were scheduled to be performed at the end of the 3rd month.

On the control visit the FEV1%, FVC%, and FEV1/FVC parameters were recorded. The asthma control status of the patients was re-assessed according to the GINA criteria and also by using the ACT. The asthma-related quality of life was re-assessed by AQLQ.

On both visits, ACT and AQLQ questionnaires were filled-in using interviewer-mediated administration technique depending on the self-reported statements of the patients.

3.3. Tools

3.3.1. Asthma Control Test [ACT]

This measure of asthma control was developed by Nathan et al. [51]. The ACT survey is a patient-completed questionnaire with 5 items assessing asthma symptoms (day- and night-time), use of rescue medications and the effect of asthma on daily functioning. All questions are scored on a 5-point Likert scale. While scoring the ACT survey, responses for each of the 5 items are summed up to yield a score ranging from 5 (poor control of asthma) to 25 (complete control of asthma) [53]. The ACT has the advantage that it does not require pulmonary function assessments. The interpretation of the questionnaire score is such that ≥20 points represent well-controlled asthma, while 16-19 points represent not well-controlled asthma and ≤15 points represent very poorly controlled asthma [48].

3.3.2. Global Initiative for Asthma [GINA] Classification

The assessment of the current clinical control status of asthma according to GINA yields three levels of asthma control described as 'controlled; partly controlled; uncontrolled' [84]. GINA classification has been shown to correlate well with the ACT-based asthma control status [83].

3.3.3. Asthma Quality of Life Questionnaire [AQLQ]

The asthma-related quality of life of the patients was assessed by the AQLQ. The AQLQ has 32 questions, 5 of which are about the patient-specific activities. At the 'initial visit', each patient was requested to select the five activities during which he/she has been most troubled by asthma during the previous 2 weeks. These activities were retained throughout the study. Patients responded to each question on a 7-point Likert scale depending on their experiences during the previous 2 weeks. Results were expressed under four domains (symptoms, 12 questions; activity limitation, 11 questions; emotional function, 5 questions; and environmental exposure, 4 questions) and as an overall score (32 questions) [76].

3.4. Statistical Analysis

Statistical analysis was performed using the commercial statistics program SPSS® 11.5. Continuous variables are presented as mean ± standard deviation (SD), while categorical variables are presented as n (%). Paired samples t-test was used to test the significance of the difference between the two visits in terms of continuous variables, while the chi-square test was used for categorical variables. The correlation between the continuous variables was tested with Pearson's correlation analysis; while the correlation between the categorical variables was tested by Spearman's correlation analysis. The relationship of the variables with the quality of life score was analyzed by univariate linear regression analysis. A p-value <0.05 within a 95% confidence interval was considered statistically significant.

4. RESULTS

4.1. General Characteristics of the Patients

The mean (standard deviation) age of the patients was 38.64 years (12.29) [range: 18-65] and 80% of the patients were women. The educational status of the patients was as shown in Figure 1. Ten percent of the patients were illiterate, while only 6% graduated from a university.

According to the National Heart Lung & Blood Institute classification, 28% of the patients were obese, 34% were overweight, 2% were thin and the rest had normal weight.

Only 4% of the patients paid their health expenditures out-of-the-pocket. State's Social Security System paid for the health expenditures of the majority (96%) of the patients.

When the heating systems used for the patients' homes were questioned, it was seen that most (62%) of the patients used natural gas, 22% used coal-burning stoves, 12% used wood-burning stoves and 4% used electrical heaters (Figure 2).

The smoking status of the patients was as presented in Table 10. Of the patients 68% stated that they never smoked, while 12% were currently smoking; the rest were ex-smokers (4% quitted smoking in the past year and 16% quitted more than a year ago). The total of the smokers and the ex-smokers were found to have smoked for a mean (SD) period of 4.63 (9.08) years and a mean (SD) number of 4.98 (10.82) cigarettes per day.

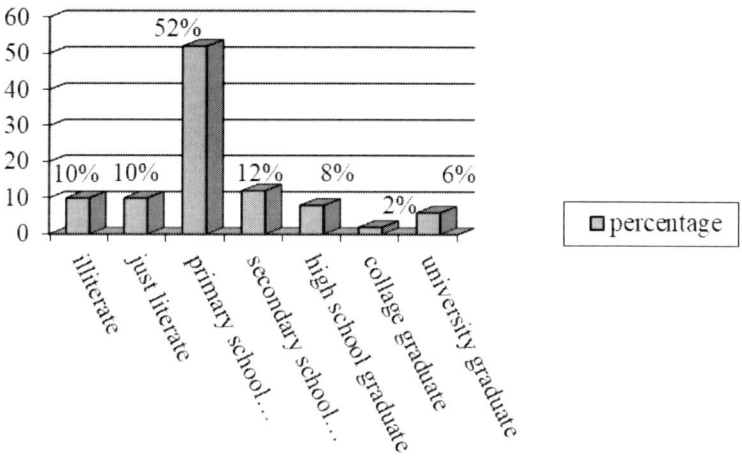

Figure 1. Educational status of the patients.

Second-hand smoking status of patients was as presented in Table 11. Forty-six percent of the patients stated that they were or had been a second-hand smoker. Two percent had been second-hand smokers at home at childhood; while, 32% were still second-hand smokers at home and 12% were current passive smokers at work.

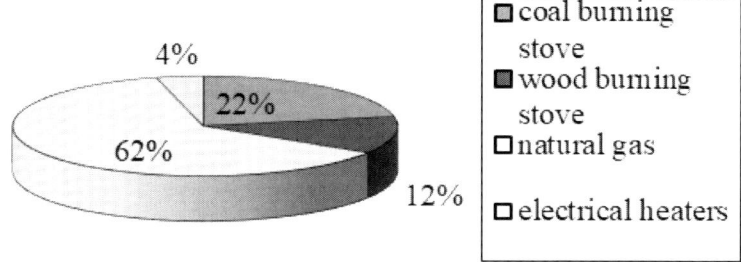

Figure 2. Heating systems used for the patients' homes.

Table 10. The smoking status of the patients

Smoking status	n	%
Never smoked	34	68
Currently smoking	6	12
Quitted smoking (more than 1 year ago)	8	16
Quitted smoking (less than 1 year)	2	4

Table 11. Second-hand smoking status of the patients

Second-hand smoking status	n	%
Non-second-hand smoker	27	54
At home	16	32
At home at childhood	1	2
At work	6	12

4.2. Clinical Features of the Patients

According to the patient records and patient self-reports, 66% of the patients had no comorbid conditions. The most frequent comorbidities were hypertension (14%) and diabetes (14%); these were followed by psychiatric disorders (4%), gastrointestinal disorders (4%), thyroid disorders (4%) and coronary artery disease (2%) (Figure 3).

The majority (92%) of the patients did not have any respiratory disease other than asthma; while 6% had chronic bronchitis and 2% had a history of tuberculosis. On the other hand, first-degree relatives of 60% of the patients were found to have asthma. The atopy status of the patients was as presented in Table 12.

The majority (96%) of the patients had no ear-nose-throat disease, while 2% had sinusitis. None of them had a history of ear-nose-throat operation.

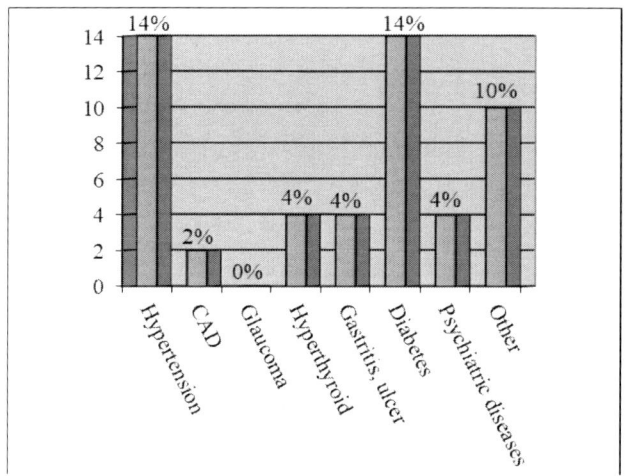

Figure 3. Comorbidities of the patients (CAD: coronary artery disease).

Table 12. Atopy status of the patients

Atopy symptoms	n	%
No atopy symptom	10	20
Skin (eczema, atopic dermatitis, redness, itching)	18	36
Nasal symptoms (occlusion, rhinitis, sneezing, itchy palate)	34	68
Conjunctivitis (eye redness and itching)	29	58
Medication allergy (penicillin group or other)	2	4
Food allergy (swelling of the tongue/lips, runny nose, shortness of breath, edema)	6	12

4.3. Asthma-Related Features of the Patients

The asthma symptoms of the patients on admission were as presented in Table 13. The majority of the patients suffered from almost all asthma symptoms.

When questioned whether the symptoms were recurrent within the day, 96% of the patients reported that their symptoms recurred during the day and 2% of the patients stated that their symptoms did not recur. The variability of symptoms during the day and night was as presented in Figure 4. The duration of the symptoms was as shown in Table 14.

Table 13. Asthma symptoms of the patients on admission

Asthma symptoms	n	%
Chest tightness	48	96
Wheezing	39	78
Cough	45	90
Phlegm/mucus	40	80
Shortness of breath	47	94

Table 14. Duration of symptoms

Duration of symptoms	n	%
≤ 1 year	11	22
> 1 year - ≤ 5 years	24	48
> 5 years - ≤ 10 years	7	14
> 10 years	8	16

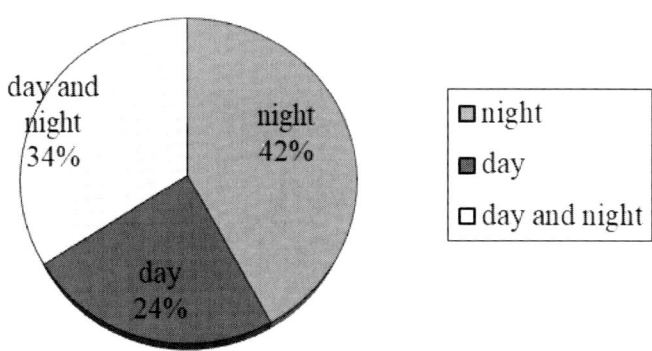

Figure 4. Variability of symptoms during day and night.

It was found that most of the patients (96%) had at least one risk factor for asthma. Asthma risk factors recorded in patients were as presented in Table 15.

Table 15. Asthma risk factors recorded in patients

Asthma risk factors	n	%
Hyperreactivity to aspirin or analgesics	3	6
Complaints when in contact with animals	6	12
Symptoms of gastroesophageal reflux (heartburn, regurgitation of food, cough, etc. worsening at night)	19	38
Increased rate of viral infections	38	76
Symptom aggravation during air pollution	39	78
None	2	4

4.4. Asthma Treatment Modalities

All patients have used inhaled corticosteroids (ICS) and/or long-acting beta2-agonists (LABA) for at least one month and short-acting beta2-agonists (SABA) when needed. The treatment modalities of the patients were as shown in Table 16. Adverse effects reported by patients at the 'final visit' are shown in Table 17.

Table 16. Treatment modalities of the patients

	n	%
High dose ICS and/or LABA	13	26
Medium dose ICS + LABA	20	40
Low dose ICS + LABA	8	16
Medium dose ICS	4	8
Low dose ICS	5	10

ICS: inhaled corticosteroid; LABA: long-acting beta2-agonist.

4.5. Pulmonary Function Parameters

The mean expected FEV1%, FEV1/FVC and FVC values recorded at the initial visit were as shown in Table 18.

4.6. Impact of Montelukast Add-On Therapy

4.6.1. Impact of Montelukast Add-On Therapy on Asthma Control Status

The effect of montelukast addition to the asthma maintenance treatment was assessed by comparing the initial asthma control status of patients with their final asthma control status. The rate of uncontrolled asthma patients assessed according to ACT score and GINA guidelines at the initial and the final visits were as shown in Figure 5. After the addition of montelukast to the treatment, the rate of uncontrolled patients decreased by 36-54%.

Table 17. Adverse effects reported by patients at the final visit

	n	Tremor (%)	Cramp, muscle pain (%)	Tachycardia (%)	Oral candidiasis (%)	Stomachache, nausea (%)	Hoarseness (%)	Other (weight gain) (%)	No adverse effect (%)
High dose ICS and LABA + M	13	0	0	15	15	0	23	8	92
Medium dose ICS and LABA + M	20	20	5	10	20	5	35	10	90
Low dose ICS and LABA + M	8	13	0	0	25	13	20	0	0
Medium dose ICS + M	4	0	0	0	0	0	25	0	0
Low dose ICS + M	5	0	0	0	20	0	40	0	0

ICS: inhaled corticosteroid; LABA: long-acting β2 agonist; M: montelukast.

Table 18. Pulmonary function parameters of the patients at the initial visit

	Mean ± SD	Minimum	Maximum
FEV_1 %	73.08 ± 14.58	39	99
FEV_1/FVC	83.42 ± 11.19	49	100
FVC%	75.72 ±14.82	39	109

SD: standard deviation; FEV: forced expiratory volume; FVC: forced vital capacity.

Table 19. Comparison of the ACT scores recorded at the initial and final visits

	ACT score (n=50)	
	Mean ± SD	Median (min-max)
Initial visit	13.54 ± 4.63[a]	13 (5-25)[b]
Final visit	19.16 ± 4.66[a]	19.5 (10-25)[b]

[a,b] p <0.05; SD: standard deviation; min: minumum; max: maximum.

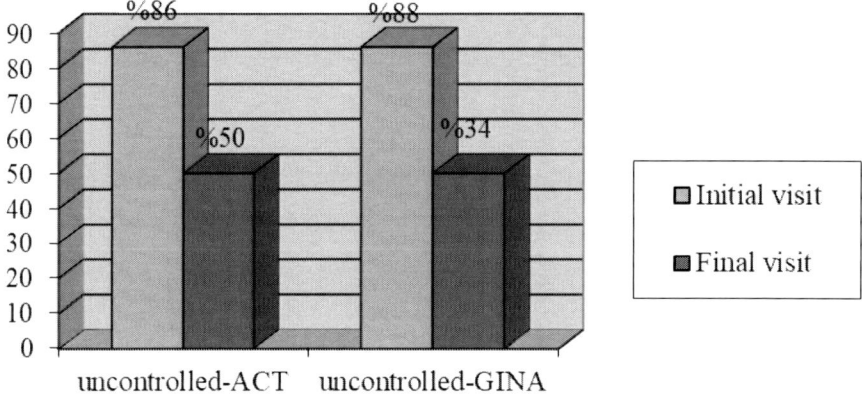

Figure 5. The rate of uncontrolled asthma patients according to ACT score and GINA guidelines at the initial and final visits.

4.6.2. Impact of Montelukast Add-On Therapy on Asthma Control Test Results

The mean and median ACT scores at the initial and final visits were as presented in Table 19. After three months of montelukast treatment, a significant increase in ACT scores was observed (p<0.05). Detailed presentation of the responses to the questions of the ACT at the initial and final visits was as presented in Table 20.

Table 20. Responses to the questions of the Asthma Control Test (n=50)

Questions	Response options	Initial visit; n (%)	Final visit; n (%)
In the past 4 weeks, how much of the time did your asthma keep you from getting as much done at work, school or at home?	All of the time	2 (4)	0 (0)
	Most of the time	14 (28)	6 (12)
	Some of the time	21 (42)	10 (20)
	A little of the time	10 (20)	17 (34)
	None of the time	3 (6)	17 (34)
During the past 4 weeks, how often have you had shortness of breath?	More than once a day	25 (50)	2 (4)
	Once a day	6 (12)	11 (22)
	3 to 6 times a week	10 (20)	8 (16)
	Once or twice a week	6 (12)	18 (36)
	Not at all	3 (6)	11 (22)
During the past 4 weeks, how often did your asthma symptoms (wheezing, coughing, shortness of breath, chest tightness or pain) wake you up at night or earlier than usual in the morning?	4 or more nights a week	9 (18)	3 (6)
	2 to 3 nights a week	15 (30)	4 (8)
	Once a week	5 (10)	2 (4)
	Once or twice	10 (20)	8 (16)
	Not at all	11 (22)	33 (66)
During the past 4 weeks, how often have you used your rescue inhaler or nebulizer medication?	3 or more times per day	12 (24)	1 (2)
	1 or 2 times per day	21 (42)	14 (28)
	2 or 3 times per week	2 (4)	6 (12)
	Once a week or less	6 (12)	6 (12)
	Not at all	9 (18)	23 (46)
How would you rate your asthma control during the past 4 weeks?	Not controlled at all	6 (12)	0 (0)
	Poorly controlled	13 (26)	9 (18)
	Somewhat controlled	16 (22)	9 (18)
	Well controlled	12 (24)	17 (34)
	Completely controlled	3 (6)	15 (30)

4.6.3. Impact of Montelukast Add-On Therapy on Asthma Control Status According to GINA Guidelines

The percentages of patients who were found to be under 'control' according to GINA guidelines at the initial and the final visits were as in Table 21. After the three months of montelukast treatment, the asthma control status of the patients according to the GINA guidelines improved significantly ($p<0.05$).

Table 21. Asthma control status according to GINA guidelines recorded at the initial and final visits (n=50)

	Controlled (%)	Partly controlled (%)	Uncontrolled (%)
Initial visit	0	14	86
Final visit	16	34	50

4.6.4. Impact of Montelukast Add-On Therapy on Spirometry Results

Mean and median values of FEV1 measurements at the initial and the final visits were as shown in Table 22. After three months of montelukast treatment, a significant improvement was observed in FEV1 values.

Table 22. Comparison of FEV1 values at the initial and final visits (n=50)

	Mean± SD	Median (min-max)
Initial visit	73.08 ± 14.58[a]	72.5 (39-99)[b]
Final visit	87.15 ± 11.31[a]	89 (47-105)[b]

[a,b] p <0.05; SD: standard deviation; min: minimum; max: maximum.

At the initial and final visits, asthma control status of the patients was determined according to the ACT score, the GINA guidelines, and the FEV1% values and expressed as 'controlled; partly controlled; uncontrolled'. The correlation among these 'asthma control statuses' determined by different parameters was tested by **Spearman's** correlation test.

At the initial visit, it was observed that ACT-based control status positively correlated with GINA-based control status (rho = 0.52; p <0.0001).

Similarly, at the final visit, it was observed that these tests still correlated with each other. ACT-based control status correlated positively with GINA-based control status (rho=0.66; p<0.0001). The asthma control status determined by FEV1 did not correlate with any of the asthma control statuses determined by the two different parameters (p>0.05). FEV1 levels alone were not sufficient to determine the status of asthma control.

4.6.5. Impact of Montelukast Add-On Therapy on Quality of Life

At the initial visit, the patients were asked to choose among the activities listed in the AQLQ, the five most challenging ones that they encountered during the last 2 weeks. The activities chosen by the patients were as shown in Table 23.

Table 23. The activities that are chosen from the AQLQ list at the initial visit

	n	%
Walking uphill/upstairs	32	64
Hurrying	30	60
Jogging/running	30	60
Housework	19	38
Sleeping	17	34
Running uphill/upstairs	14	28
Mopping or scrubbing the ground	12	24
Playing with children	12	24
Exercising/playing sports	11	22
Laughing	11	22
Talking	11	22
Walking/going for a walk	11	22
Home maintenance	9	18
Vacuuming	8	16
Carrying out activities at work	8	16
Sexual intercourse	4	8
Playing with pets	3	6
Social activities/visiting friends or relatives	3	6
Performing woodworking or carpentry	2	4
Dancing	2	4
Bicycling	1	2

The results of the AQLQ recorded at the initial and the final visits were as presented in Figure 6. The mean scores for the overall AQLQ questionnaire and for each domain (symptoms, activity limitation, emotional function, and environmental exposure) were calculated separately.

Improvement in asthma-related quality of life was found to be clinically significant as the domain scores and the overall score improved more than 0.5 points [81, 82].

Linear regression analysis was performed to investigate the effects of FEV1% and asthma control statuses determined by ACT and GINA guidelines as well as according to FEV1 level on the total and domain scores of the AQLQ.

The regression of the total and domain scores of the AQLQ at the initial visit with the asthma control status related parameters was as presented in Table 24. It was observed that the FEV1% level and the asthma control status determined according to FEV1% had no effect on AQLQ total and domain scores. On the other hand, asthma control statuses determined according to the ACT score and GINA guidelines were found to be predictive of the overall and the domain-specific asthma-related quality of life of the patients at the initial visit.

Table 24. Regression of FEV1% level and asthma control status determined according to various criteria with the total and domain scores of the AQLQ at the initial visit (n=50)

			FEV1%	Asthma control status based on		
				FEV1%	ACT	GINA
AQLQ Domains	Total	B	[-] 0.012	0.094	0.171	[-] 1.363
		SE	0.010	0.228	0.021	0.385
		P	NS	NS	0.000	0.001
	Activity limitation	B	[-] 0.014	0.152	0.150	[-] 1.169
		SE	0.011	0.234	0.026	0.413
		P	NS	NS	0.000	0.007
	Symptoms	B	[-] 0.012	0.097	0.211	[-] 1.819
		SE	0.012	0.270	0.024	0.440
		P	NS	NS	0.000	0.000
	Emotional function	B	[-] 0.007	[-] 0.048	0.172	[-] 1.156
		SE	0.013	0.287	0.033	0.517
		P	NS	NS	0.000	0.030
	Environmental exposure	B	[-] 0.010	0.107	0.109	[-] 0.792
		SE	0.011	0.254	0.033	0.468
		P	NS	NS	0.000	NS

SE: Standard error; NS: not significant, B shows the strength of the relation. [-] indicates that the regression between the dependent and the independent variable is in the opposite direction.

Table 25. Regression of FEV1% level and asthma control status determined according to various criteria with the total and domain scores of the AQLQ at the final visit (n=50)

			FEV1%	Asthma control status based on		
				FEV1%	ACT	GINA
AQLQ Domains	Total	B	0.035	[-] 0.643	0.188	[-] 0.889
		SE	0.014	0.337	0.023	0.183
		P	0.015	NS	0.000	0.000
	Activity limitation	B	0.027	[-] 0.393	0.180	[-] 0.838
		SE	0.016	0.384	0.030	0.217
		P	NS	NS	0.000	0.000
	Symptoms	B	0.044	[-] 0.815	0.222	[-] 1.016
		SE	0.015	0.359	0.022	0.192
		P	0.004	0.028	0.000	0.000
	Emotional function	B	0.048	[-] 1.188	0.187	[-] 0.964
		SE	0.18	0.417	0.037	0.252
		P	0.010	0.006	0.000	0.000
	Environmental exposure	B	0.014	[-] 0.133	0.114	[-] 0.558
		SE	0.018	0.428	0.041	0.262
		P	NS	NS	0.007	0.038

SE: Standard error; NS: not significant, B shows the strength of the relation. [-] indicates that the regression between the dependent and the independent variable is in the opposite direction.

The regression of the total and domain scores of the AQLQ at the final visit with the asthma control status related parameters was as presented in Table 25. It was observed that asthma control status determined according to FEV1% had no effect on AQLQ total score. On the other hand, asthma control statuses determined according to the ACT score and GINA guidelines were found to be predictive of the overall and the domain-specific asthma-related quality of life of the patients at the final visit.

The correlation of the ACT score with the total and domain scores of the AQLQ at the initial visit was as presented in Table 26. ACT score correlated significantly with the total and domain scores of the AQLQ ($p<0.05$).

The correlation of the ACT score with the total and domain scores of the AQLQ at the final visit was as presented in Table 27. ACT score correlated significantly with the total and domain scores of the AQLQ ($p<0.05$).

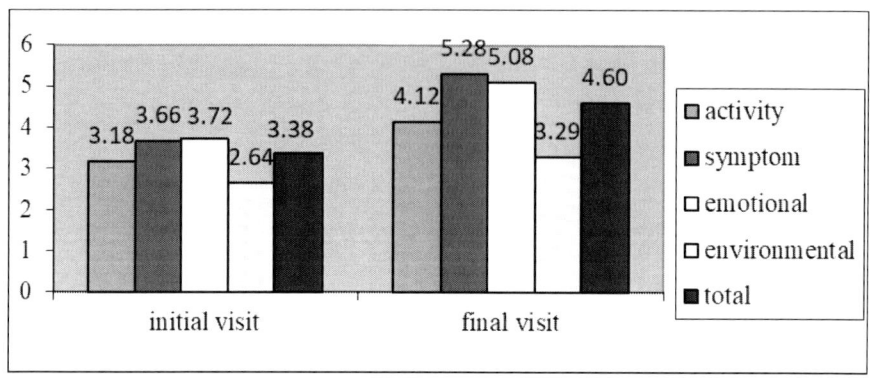

Figure 6. Total score and domain (symptoms, activity limitation, emotional function and environmental exposure) scores of the AQLQ.

Table 26. Correlation of the ACT score with the total and domain scores of the AQLQ at the initial visit

	AQLQ total, rho	AQLQ act, rho	AQLQ sym, rho	AQLQ emo, rho	AQLQ env, rho
ACT score	.713[a]	-.600[a]	.758[a]	.558[a]	.365[b]

[a]$p< 0.0001$; [b]$p<0.01$; rho: Spearman's rho correlation coefficient, act: activity limitation, sym: symptoms, emo: emotional function, env: environmental exposure.

Table 27. Correlation of the ACT score with the total and domain scores of the AQLQ at the final visit

	AQLQ total, rho	AQLQ act, rho	AQLQ sym, rho	AQLQ emo, rho	AQLQ env, rho
ACT score	.729[a]	.627[a]	.771[a]	.559[a]	.322[b]

[a]$p< 0.0001$; [b]$p<0.05$; rho: Spearman's rho correlation coefficient, act: activity limitation, sym: symptoms, emo: emotional function, env: environmental exposure.

5. DISCUSSION

Leukotriene receptor antagonists have various effects on asthma. Montelukast as add-on therapy administered to asthma patients using high dose corticosteroids was found to have positive effects on symptom scores when compared with placebo at 3 and 12 weeks [85]. In our study, we aimed to assess the effect of the leukotriene receptor antagonist montelukast as add-on therapy on symptom control and quality of life of asthma patients.

Montelukast add-on therapy administered for three months resulted in improvements in asthma control status assessed by two different asthma control scales/criteria, namely the ACT scale and the GINA criteria.

At a study conducted on 191 asthma patients, Tohda et al. [86] found out that daily administration of 10 mg montelukast decreased the need for moderate and high dose inhaled corticosteroids in clinically stable patients. Similarly, Laviolette et al. [87] reported that leukotriene receptor antagonist addition to uncontrolled asthma patients receiving inhaled corticosteroids helped asthma be under control.

Patients in our study were using long-acting beta2-agonists alone or in combination with an inhaled corticosteroid for at least one month before montelukast prescription. The general approach in asthma treatment is gradually increasing the inhaled corticosteroid doses. Coutts et al. [88] reported that montelukast was the most appropriate leukotriene receptor antagonist improving treatment with long-term inhaled corticosteroids. In addition, for the non-adherent patients, montelukast had the advantage that it can be dosed only once daily [88].

In other efficacy studies conducted on asthma patients, leukotriene receptor antagonists were shown to be much less effective (but much more expensive) than inhaled corticosteroids [89]. Leukotriene receptor antagonists are used in mild asthma as add-on or prophylactic treatment in patients receiving inhaled beta2-agonists and corticosteroids [90].

In some studies, 7-28% of patients started to use an LTRA at their first visit [91, 92]. According to Juniper's ACQ survey, 79% of asthma patients were not well controlled at the first visit and 83% of them used LTRA as mono or combination therapy with inhalation therapies.

Combinations of steroids and long-acting beta2-agonists also improve pulmonary parameters in asthma patients. However, beta2-agonists have no anti-inflammatory effects. In many studies, it has been shown that montelukast yields anti-inflammatory effects in asthma patients by decreasing the number of eosinophils in blood and sputum [93].

Leukotriene receptor antagonists reduce airway inflammation associated with allergen-induced airway response [94]. Many placebo-controlled studies have shown that the eosinophil count was a marker of inflammation and treatment with leukotriene receptor antagonists significantly reduced the eosinophil counts [85, 95].

In a 12-week comparative study by Ringdal et al. [96], patients using salmeterol and fluticasone propionate were found to be more satisfied with the treatment than those using fluticasone propionate and montelukast, and the physicians who prescribed the treatment found this treatment more beneficial ($p<0.05$).

Wilson et al. at their three parallel group study prescribed the patients who were receiving inhaled corticosteroids, one of the three medications: montelukast, zafirlukast, and salmeterol. They observed that salmeterol improved pulmonary function more than the other drugs and decreased asthma symptoms more [97].

Asthma treatment is supposed to improve airway inflammation, respiratory function, and symptoms. The level of asthma control is determined by the frequency and intensity of symptoms, pulmonary function test values, daily bronchodilator drug need to relieve symptoms and limitation of physical activities [98]. Completely controlled asthma patients should not have daytime/night symptoms, activity limitations, any asthma attack and need for rescue/relief medications and their respiratory functions (PEF, FEV1) should be normal [9]. The main purpose of asthma treatment is to control the disease by reducing symptoms and attacks and improving respiratory function [8]. In our study, we assessed the asthma control levels of the patients using the validated Turkish version of the ACT questionnaire.

In our study, it was observed that GINA-based asthma control status positively correlated with ACT-based asthma control status (rho=0.52; $p<0.0001$). At a multi-center study, El-Hasnaoui et al. [99] observed a similar positive correlation between the asthma control status defined according to the GINA criteria and the ACT scores.

In our study, ACT scores and FEV1% were not correlated with each other. Similar to our results, at a study conducted on 313 patients Schatz et al. [53] found a weaker correlation between ACT scores and FEV1% (r=0.29, p<0.001).

In this present study, montelukast addition to the therapy resulted in a significant decrease in beta2-agonist use. This finding is in accordance with the results of other studies in the literature. Virchow et al. [100] reported a decrease in beta2-agonist use and improvement of asthma symptoms as a consequence of montelukast addition to therapy. Likewise, Samarzija et al. [101] observed significant improvements in FEV1 values and clinical conditions of the patients, as well as a significant decrease in salbutamol use as a result of adding montelukast to current therapies of a population of 612 patients.

The mean (SD) FEV1% value, which was initially 73.08 (14.58) increased to 87.15 (11.31) after the addition of montelukast to the therapy (p<0.0001). Similar to our results, Virchow et al. [102] reported a smaller increase in FEV1% levels [from 79.2 (21.2) to 84 (22.2)] as a result of 3-month montelukast add-on therapy (p<0.0001). At a randomized single-blinded controlled trial on acute asthma attacks, 10 mg oral montelukast was given to the treatment group as add-on to standard therapy for 2 weeks [103]. It was stated that the montelukast group had better peak expiratory flow rate (PEFR) at 2 and 4 weeks (p<0.0376 and p<0.0003 respectively) and had a better FEV1 value at the end of 4 weeks (p<0.0033) as compared to the control group. Another study indicated that add-on montelukast therapy to standard therapy had no beneficial effect on acute asthma attacks [104].

In the majority of our patients, asthma was not under control despite the utilization of combination drug therapies. At their study conducted on a total of 1681 patients, Virchow et al. [102] identified that 23.1% of the patients were using inhaled corticosteroids alone, while, 69.5% were using LABAs alone or in combination; and despite these therapies, asthma was noted to be inadequately controlled.

The reasons for the uncontrolled asthma despite the therapy could be active or second-hand smoking, respiratory tract infections, acute or chronic allergen exposition, and other factors (obesity, gastroesophageal reflux disease, various nasal and sinus diseases, inappropriate drug use such as beta-blockers, air pollution, hormonal changes, psychological disorders, etc.) [105]. Inadequate benefit from the medications could also be a consequence of the patients' nonadherence to therapy and failing to use the inhaler devices by the proper technique.

The mean (SD) ACT score, which was initially 13.54 (4.63) increased to 19.16 (4.66) after the addition of montelukast to the therapy (p<0.0001). Virchow et al. [102] reported a similar increase in ACT score [from 14.6 (4.6) to 18.8 (4.4)] as a result of 3-month montelukast add-on therapy (p<0.0001). However, another study by Baig et al. [106] stated that montelukast did not have any significant impact on the ACT score.

At the beginning of the study, asthma was completely controlled in only 4% of the patients (whose ACT score was 25); this rate increased to 16% after 3-month montelukast add-on therapy. Virchow at al. [102] reported more modest results where the rate of fully controlled patients, which was 1.2% initially, increased to 11.4% after 6-month montelukast therapy.

FitzGerald et al. [107] reported improvements in asthma control as a result of montelukast addition to the therapies of the patients who were receiving corticosteroids alone.

In their study conducted in asthma patients over 15 years of age, Dupont et al. [108] recorded significant improvements in ACQ scores after treatment with montelukast for two months. They also recorded a significant decrease in the requirement of rescue (reliever) medications and an improvement in respiratory functions (p<0.001).

Noonan et al. [109] conducted a study on patients with mild and moderate asthma and observed significant dose-related improvements in asthma control (as assessed by FEV1 and PEF values, and daytime symptom scores) with the addition of montelukast to their current therapies. In addition, asthma-specific quality of life was improved, and the daily requirement of inhaled β2-agonists was decreased. After 2-week montelukast treatment 78.6% of the patients improved, while 20.7% had no change and 0.7% got worse [109].

Asthma is a chronic disease affecting the patients' lives physically, emotionally and socially and when it is uncontrolled it leads to a decrease in productivity as well as the quality of life of the patients [7]. In recent years, quality of life assessments are getting more important as a way to evaluate this aspect of the disease. Therefore, we assessed the quality of life status of our patients using the Asthma Quality of Life Questionnaire (AQLQ) which is an asthma-specific questionnaire developed by Juniper et al. [76].

Juniper et al. [76] reported that AQLQ is a valid questionnaire for the evaluation of the quality of life in asthma patients and is sensitive to detect asthma-related changes in the quality of life of the patients. The Turkish version of the AQLQ was validated in Turkish asthma patients by Sahin et al. [110].

In our study, the mean (SD) AQLQ score which was initially 3.4 (1.0) increased to 4.6 (1.2) after 3-month montelukast add-on therapy.

Montelukast treatment resulted in significant improvement in the overall AQLQ scale as well as in activity limitation, symptoms, emotional function and environmental exposure scales.

Our results were in accordance with those of Virchow et al. [102] where the effect of montelukast addition to current therapy on patients' quality of life was assessed using the short version of AQLQ (mini-AQLQ). That study yielded significant improvements in all four scales of the AQLQ as a consequence of montelukast add-on therapy ($p<0.0001$; for all).

In a double-blind randomized control trial with 156 patients, Baig et al. [106] reported that the mean ± SD of total QOL on AQLQ-S increased from 3.74±0.88 to 5.06±0.89 for montelukast group and from 3.58±0.92 to 4.71±0.97 for the placebo group ($p=0.02$) after 4 weeks add-on therapy. The study also indicated that significant improvement was observed only environmental scale with 5.06±0.89 for the montelukast group and 4.71±0.97 for the placebo group ($p=0.02$).

Different results were obtained at studies done by using AQLQ. In a study, there was no difference in terms of any AQLQ-scale scores between patients using fluticasone propionate and leukotriene receptor antagonists;

while with only fluticasone propionate significant difference was observed in symptom and emotional function scales. In a study with 20 mg zafirlukast twice a day, it was found that there was no significant superiority compared to placebo [111].

Hubert et al. [112] observed that asthma control the most strongly correlated with activity scale (r=0.50, p<0.0001) and the weakly correlated with environmental scale (r=0.37, p<0.0001).

In our study AQLQ was shown to be correlated with GINA and ACT; therefore, improvement in asthma control status results in the improvement in AQLQ. Similarly, Chhabra and Kaushik [113] found a positive correlation between total AQLQ score and ACQ score (r=0.522), a stronger correlation was observed between the AQLQ-symptom domain score and ACQ score (r=0.631). However, they failed to find a correlation between FEV1% and AQLQ total score and other AQLQ-scale scores. AQLQ represents the patient's quality of life in the last 15 days; therefore, it may not be well correlated with parameters of respiratory function.

When its effects on asthma control status, quality of life and respiratory functions are considered, montelukast addition to ongoing asthma treatment with LABA and/or inhaled steroids seems to be beneficiary.

CONCLUSION

There is sufficient evidence that asthma can be controlled by appropriate treatment. Pharmacological treatment can improve symptoms, prevent, reduce the frequency and severity of exacerbations, and increase exercise tolerance. Thus, increases the quality of life. As a result, considering the effects of patients on asthma control status, quality of life and pulmonary function, it was seen that adding montelukast to the treatment of asthma with LABA and/or inhaled steroids is a useful approach.

REFERENCES

[1] Gemicioğlu, Bilun. 2001. "Bronş Astımı" [Bronchial asthma]. In *Göğüs Hastalıkları II. Cilt*, 619-661. Istanbul: Santay Matbaacılık.

[2] Centers for Disease Control and Prevention. 2019. "*Asthma.*" Accessed March 28. https://www.cdc.gov/asthma/default.htm.

[3] Centers for Disease Control and Prevention. 2019. "*Asthma Surveillance Data.*" 2019. Accessed March 28. https://www.cdc.gov/asthma/asthmadata.htm.

[4] Centers for Disease Control and Prevention. 2019. "*Most Recent Asthma Data Available From CDC.*" Accessed March 28. https://www.cdc.gov/asthma/most_recent_data.htm.

[5] The Global Asthma Network. 2018. "*Global Asthma Report 2018.*" Auckland, New Zealand: The Global Asthma Network. http://www.globalasthmareport.org/.

[6] Beyhun, N. Ercüment, and Nesrin Çilingiroğlu. 2004. "Hastalık Maliyeti ve Astım." ["Cost of Diseases and Asthma."]. *Tüberküloz Ve Toraks* 52(4):386-392.

[7] Yakar, Tansu, Ateş Baran, Murat Yalçınsoy, Onur Çelik, Sinem Güngör, Günay Can, and Esen Akkaya. 2006. "Astımlı Hastalarda Yaşam Kalitesinin Belirlenmesi." ["Assessment of Quality of Life in Asthma Patients"]. *İzmir Göğüs Hastalıkları Dergisi* 20(1):1-10.

[8] Yorgancıoğlu, Arzu. 2000. "Astım Tedavisinde Yenilikler ve Lökotrien Antagonistleri." ["Updates in Asthma Treatment and Leukotriene Antagonsits."] *Toraks Dergisi* 1(2):58-68.

[9] Türk Toraks Derneği. 2009 "Astım Tanı Ve Tedavi Rehberi." ["Turkish Thoracic Society – Guidelines for the Diagnosis and Treatment of Asthma."]. *Turkish Thoracic Journal* 10(10):1-75.

[10] Sorkness, Christine A., and Kathryn V. Blake. 2017. "Asthma." In *Pharmacotherapy: A Pathophysiologic Approach, 10e,* edited by Joseph T. DiPiro, Robert L. Talbert, Gary C. Yee, Gary R. Matzke, Barbara G. Wells, and L. Michael Posey. New York: McGraw-Hill.

[11] Global Initiative for Asthma. 2006. "*Global Strategy for Asthma Management and Prevention.*" https://ginasthma.org/archived-reports/.
[12] Sorkness, Christine A. 2001. "Leukotriene Receptor Antagonists in the Treatment of Asthma." *Pharmacotherapy* 21(3 Part 2):34S-37S.
[13] Sheth, Ketan, Rohit Borker, Amanda Emmett, Kathleen Rickard, and Paul Dorinsky. 2002. "Cost-Effectiveness Comparison of Salmeterol/Fluticasone Propionate versus Montelukast in the Treatment of Adults with Persistent Asthma." *Pharmacoeconomics* 20(13):909-918.
[14] Romagnoli, Micaela, Luca Richeldi, and Leonardo M. Fabbri. 2002. "Clinical Assessment of Asthma and COPD: Diagnosis." In *Asthma and COPD*, edited by Peter Barnes, Jeffrey Drazen, Stephen Rennard, and Neil Thomson, 447-455. London: Academic Press.
[15] Bousquet, Jean, Peter K. Jeffery, William W. Busse, Malcolm Johnson, and Antonio M. Vignola. 2000. "Asthma. From Bronchoconstriction to Airways Inflammationand Remodelling." *American Journal Of Respiratory And Critical Care Medicine* 161(5):1720-1745.
[16] Havluvu, Yavuz. 2006. *Astımlı Olgularda İnflamasyon Takibinde Yüksek Rezolüsyonlu Bilgisayarlı Tomografinin Yerinin ve Lökotrien Reseptör Antagonistlerinin İnflamasyona olan Etkisinin Değerlendirilmesi. [Assessment of the Role of High Resolution Computed Tomography in Monitoring Inflammation and the Evaluation of Influence of Leukotriene Receptor Antagonists on Inflammation in Patients with Asthma]*. PhD diss., Celal Bayar University, Faculty of Medicine, Department of Chest Diseases
[17] Scott T. Weiss. 1998. "Asthma: Epidemiology." In *Fishman's Pulmonary Diseases and Disorders, 3e*, edited by Altred P. Fishman, Jack A. Elias, Jay A. Fishman, Michael A. Grippi, Larry R. Kaiser, and Robert M. Senior, 735-43. McGraw-Hill.
[18] Öneş, Ülker, Nihat Sapan, Ayper Somer, Rian Dişçi, Nuran Salman, Nermin Güler, and Işık Yalçın. 1997. "Prevalence of Childhood Asthma in Istanbul, Turkey." *Allergy* 52(5):570-575.

[19] Selçuk, Ziya Toros, Tuncay Çağlar, Tayfun Enünlü, and Tuğba Topal. 1997. "The Prevalence of Allergic Diseases in Primary School Children in Edirne, Turkey." *Clinical & Experimental Allergy* 27(3):262-269.

[20] Tarraf, Hesham, Omur Aydin, Dilsad Mungan, Mohammad Albader, Bassam Mahboub, Adam Doble, Aaicha *Lahlou, Luqman Tariq, Fayaz* Aziz, and Abdelkader El Hasnaoui. 2018. "Prevalence of Asthma among the Adult General Population of Five Middle Eastern Countries: Results of the SNAPSHOT Program." *BMC Pulmonary Medicine* 18(1):68.

[21] Türk Toraks Derneği. 2016. *"Türk Toraks Derneği Astım Tanı Ve Tedavi Rehberi 2016."* [*"Turkish Thoracic Society – Guidelines for the Diagnosis and Treatment of Asthma 2016."*]. Ankara, Turkey: Türk Toraks Derneği. https://www.toraks.org.tr/book.aspx?list=2212&menu=288

[22] Centers for Disease Control and Prevention. 1995. "Asthma-United States, 1982-1992." *JAMA: The Journal of the American Medical Association* 273(6):451-452.

[23] Weiss, Kevin B., Peter J. Gergen, and Thomas A. Hodgson. 1992. "An Economic Evaluation of Asthma in the United States." *New England Journal of Medicine* 326(13):862-866.

[24] Küçükusta, Ahmet Rasim. 2005. "Epidemiyoloji." ["Epidemiology."]. In *Tanıdan Tedaviye Astım*, edited by Bilun Gemicioğlu, 5-26. Istanbul: Turgut Yayıncılık ve Ticaret A.S.

[25] D'Amato, Gennaro, Carolina Vitale, Antonio Molino, Anna Stanziola, Alessandro Sanduzzi, Alessandro Vatrella, Mauro Mormile, Maurizia Lanza, Giovanna Calabrese, Leonardo Antonicelli, and Maria D'Amato. 2016. "Asthma-Related Deaths." *Multidisciplinary Respiratory Medicine* 11:37.

[26] Global Initiative for Asthma. 2018. *"Global Strategy for Asthma Management and Prevention."* https://ginasthma.org/gina-reports/.

[27] Cookson, William O. C. M., Jennifer A. Faux, Pamela A. Sharp, and Julian M. Hopkin. 1989. "Linkage between Immunoglobulin E

Responses Underlying Asthma and Rhinitis and Chromosome 11q." *The Lancet* 333(8650):1292-1295.
[28] Duffy, David L., Charles A. Mitchell, and Nicholas G. Martin. 1998. "Genetic and Environmental Risk Factors for Asthma." *American Journal of Respiratory and Critical Care Medicine* 157(3):840-845.
[29] Doğan, İsmail. 2008. *Astım Kontrolünün Değerlendirilmesinde Astım Kontrol Testi ve Fraksiyone Ekshale Nitrik Oksitin Yeri*. [*Role of Asthma Control Test and Fractioned Exhaled Nitric Oxide for the Assessment of Asthma Control Status*]. PhD diss., Istanbul University, Cerrahpaşa Medicine Faculty, Department of Chest Diseases.
[30] Niimi, Akio, Hisako Matsumoto, Ryoichi Amitani, Yasutaka Nakano, Michiaki Mishima, Masayoshi Minakuchi, Koichi Nishimura, Harumi Itoh, and Takateru Izumi. 2000. "Airway Wall Thickness in Asthma Assessed by Computed Tomography." *American Journal of Respiratory and Critical Care Medicine* 162(4):1518-1523.
[31] Bergeron, Céline, Meri K. Tulic, and Qutayba Hamid. 2010. "Airway remodelling in asthma: From benchside to clinical practice." *Can Respir J*. 17(4):e85–e93.
[32] Masoli, Matthew, Denise Fabian, Shaun Holt, and Richard Beasley. 2004. "The Global Burden Of Asthma: Executive Summary of the GINA Dissemination Committee Report." *Allergy* 59(5):469-478.
[33] Ishmael, Faoud T. 2011. "The Inflammatory Response in the Pathogenesis of Asthma." *The Journal of the American Osteopathic Association* 111:S11-S17.
[34] Türktaş, Haluk. 2005. "Astım." ["Asthma"]. *Toraks Derneği* 4. Kış Okulu, Kayseri, Ocak 4-8.
[35] Sibbald, Bonnie, Mary E. C. Horn, and Ian Gregg. 1980. "A Family Study of the Genetic Basis of Asthma and Wheezy Bronchitis." *Archives of Disease in Childhood* 55(5):354-357.
[36] Holloway, John W., Bianca Beghé, and Stephen T. Holgate. 1999. "The Genetic Basis of Atopic Asthma." *Clinical Experimental Allergy* 29(8):1023-032.

[37] Pearce, Neil, Juha Pekkanen, and Richard Beasley. 1999. "How Much Asthma is Really Attributable to Atopy?" *Thorax* 54(3):268-272.

[38] Martinez, Fernando D. 2000. "Viruses and Atopic Sensitization in the First Years of Life." *American Journal of Respiratory and Critical Care Medicine* 162(supplement_2):S95-S99.

[39] Laprise, Catherine, and Louis-Philippe Boulet. 1997. "Asymptomatic Airway Hyperresponsiveness: A Three-Year Follow-Up." *American Journal of Respiratory and Critical Care Medicine* 156(2):403-409.

[40] Le Souef, Peter N. 1993. In *Expression of Predisposing Factors in Early Life: Asthma Physiology, Immunopharmacology and Treatment,* edited by Stephen T. Holgate, 41-60. London: Academic Press.

[41] Pearce, Neil, Jeroen Douwes, and Richard Beasley. 2000. "Is Allergen Exposure the Major Primary Cause of Asthma?" *Thorax* 55(5):424-431.

[42] Rasanen, M., T. Laitinen, J. Kaprıo, M. Koskenvuo, and L. A. Laitinen. 1997. "Hay Fever, Asthma and Number of Older Siblings - A Twin Study." *Clinical Experimental Allergy* 27(5):515-518.

[43] British Thoracic Society. 2008. "British Guideline on the Management of Asthma." *Thorax* 63(Supplement 4):iv1-iv121.

[44] Vollmer, William M., Leona E. Markson, Elizabeth O'connor, Lesly L. Sanocki, Leslye Fitterman, Marc Berger, and A. Sonia Buist. 1999. "Association of Asthma Control with Health Care Utilization and Quality of Life." *American Journal of Respiratory and Critical Care Medicine* 160(5 Pt 1):1647-1652.

[45] Türk Toraks Derneği. 2014. "*Türk Toraks Derneği Astım Tanı Ve Tedavi Rehberi 2014.*" ["*Turkish Thoracic Society – Guidelines for the Diagnosis and Treatment of Asthma 2014.*"]. Ankara, Turkey: Türk Toraks Derneği. https://www.toraks.org.tr/book.aspx?list=1695&menu=242.

[46] National Asthma Education and Prevention Program. 2007. "Expert Panel Report 3 (EPR-3): Guidelines for the Diagnosis and

Management of Asthma–Summary Report 2007." *Journal of Allergy and Clinical Immunology* 120(5):S94-S138.

[47] Asthma Therapy Assessment Questionnaire (ATAQ). In. *West Point*. Pensylvania: Merck & Co Inc, 1997–1999.

[48] Juniper, Elizabeth F., Paul M. O′Byrne, Gordon H. Guyatt, Penelope J. Ferrie, and Derek R. King. 1999. "Development and Validation of a Questionnaire to Measure Asthma Control." *European Respiratory Journal* 14(4):902.

[49] Ehrs, Per-Olof, Mika Nokela, Björn Ställberg, Paul Hjemdahl, and Eva Wikström Jonsson. 2006. "Brief Questionnaires for Patient-Reported Outcomes in Asthma: Validation and Usefulness in a Primary Care Setting." *Chest* 129(4):925-932.

[50] Boulet, Louis-Philippe, Véronique Boulet, and Joanne Milot. 2002. "How Should We Quantify Asthma Control? A Proposal." *Chest* 122 (6): 2217-2223.

[51] Nathan, Robert A., Christine A. Sorkness, Mark Kosinski, Michael Schatz, James T. Li, Philip Marcus, John J. Murray, and Trudy B. Pendergraft. 2004. "Development of the Asthma Control Test: A Survey for Assessing Asthma Control." *Journal of Allergy and Clinical Immunology* 113(1):59-65.

[52] Schatz, Michael, Robert S. Zeiger, Alexandra Drane, Kathleen Harden, Aysel Cibildak, Jon E. Oosterman, and Mark Kosinski. 2007. "Reliability and Predictive Validity of the Asthma Control Test Administered by Telephone Calls Using Speech Recognition Technology." *Journal of Allergy and Clinical Immunology* 119(2): 336-343.

[53] Schatz, Michael, Christine A. Sorkness, James T. Li, Philip Marcus, John J. Murray, Robert A. Nathan, Mark Kosinski, Trudy B. Pendergraft, and Priti Jhingran. 2006. "Asthma Control Test: Reliability, Validity, and Responsiveness in Patients Not Previously Followed By Asthma Specialists." *Journal Of Allergy And Clinical Immunology* 117(3):549-556.

[54] Abadoğlu, Öznur. 2008. "Astım kontrolünün değerlendirme anketleri." ["Questionnaires for the Assessment of Asthma Control."]. *Asthma Allergy Immunol* 6(2):99-104.

[55] Newman, Stephen P. 2005. "Inhaler Treatment Options In COPD." *European Respiratory Review* 14(96):102-108.

[56] Juniper, Elizabeth F., Patricia A. Kline, Michael A. Vanzieleghem, E. Helen Ramsdale, Paul M. O'byrne, and Frederick E. Hargreave. 1990. "Effect of Long-Term Treatment with an Inhaled Corticosteroid (Budesonide) on Airway Hyperresponsiveness and Clinical Asthma in Nonsteroid-Dependent Asthmatics." *American Review Of Respiratory Disease* 142(4):832-836.

[57] Pauwels, Romain A., Claes-Göran Löfdahl, Dirkje S. Postma, Anne E. Tattersfield, Paul O'Byrne, Peter J. Barnes, and Anders Ullman. 1997. "Effect of Inhaled Formoterol and Budesonide on Exacerbations of Asthma." *New England Journal of Medicine* 337(20):1405-1411.

[58] Gibson, Peter G., Heather Powell, and Francine M. Ducharme. 2007. "Differential Effects of Maintenance Long-Acting B-Agonist and Inhaled Corticosteroid on Asthma Control and Asthma Exacerbations." *Journal of Allergy and Clinical Immunology* 119(2): 344-350.

[59] Rabe, Klaus F., Emilio Pizzichini, Björn Ställberg, Santiago Romero, Ana M. Balanzat, Tito Atienza, Per Arve Lier, and Carin Jorup. 2006. "Budesonide/Formoterol in a Single Inhaler for Maintenance and Relief in Mild-to-Moderate Asthma." *Chest* 129(2):246-256.

[60] Pauwels, Romain A., A. Sonia Buist, Peter M. A. Calverley, Christine R. Jenkins, and Suzanne S. Hurd. 2001. "Global Strategy for the Diagnosis, Management, and Prevention of Chronic Obstructive Pulmonary Disease." *American Journal of Respiratory and Critical Care Medicine* 163(5):1256-1276.

[61] Knapp, Howard R., and John J. Murray. 1994. "Leukotrienes as Mediators of Nasal Inflammation." *Adv Prostaglandin Thromboxane Leukot Res.* 22:279-288.

[62] Lipworth, Brian J. 1999. "Leukotriene-Receptor Antagonists." *The Lancet* 353(9146):57-62.

[63] Gemicioğlu, Bilun. 2004. *Tanımdan Tedaviye Astım*. [*Asthma from Identification to Treatment*]. Istanbul.

[64] Aubier, Michel, and Charis Roussos. 1985. "Effect of Theophylline on Respiratory Muscle Function." *Chest* 88(2):S91-97.

[65] Taylor, D. Robin, Brian Buick, Charles Kinney, Roger C. Lowry, and Denis G. McDevitt. 1985. "The Efficacy of Orally Administered Theophylline, Inhaled Salbutamol, and a Combination of the Two as Chronic Therapy in the Management of Chronic Bronchitis with Reversible Air-Flow Obstruction." *American Review of Respiratory Disease* 131(5):747-51.

[66] Celli, B.R., W. MacNee, A. Agusti, A. Anzueto, B. Berg, A.S. Buist, and P.M.A. Calverley et al. 2004. "Standards for the Diagnosis and Treatment of Patients with COPD: A Summary of the ATS/ERS Position Paper." *European Respiratory Journal* 23(6):932-946.

[67] Lacy, Charles F, Lora L Armstrong, Morton P Goldman, and Leonard L Lance. 2001. *Drug Information Handbook*. 9th ed. Hudson, OH: Lexi-Comp Inc.

[68] Mete, Emin, and Halil Değirmencioğlu. 2005. "Çocukluk çağı astımının güncel tedavisi ve yeni gelismeler." ["Updated treatment approach to childhood asthma and recent advances."] *C. Ü. Tıp Fakültesi Dergisi* 27(1):39-46.

[69] Solomon, William R., and Thomas A. E. Platts-Mills. 1998. Aerobiology and inhalant allergens. In: *Allergy: Principles & Practice, Volume II. 5th ed.* edited by Elliott Middleton Jr., Charles E. Reed, Elliot F. Ellis, N. Franklin Adkinson Jr., John W. Yunginger, and William W. Busse, 367-403. St Louis, Missouri: Mosby-Year Book Inc.

[70] Arslantaş, Didem, Selma Metintaş, Alaettin Ünsal, and Cemalettin Kalyoncu. 2006. "Eskişehir Mahmudiye ilçesi yaşlılarında yaşam kalitesi." ["Quality of life of the elderly residents of the Mahmudiye District of Eskişehir."]. *Osmangazi Tıp Dergisi* 28(2):81-89.

[71] Telatar, Tahsin Gökhan, and Hilal Özcebe. 2004. "Geriatrik yaşam kalitesi, Yaşlı nüfus ve yaşam kalitelerinin yükseltilmesi." ["Geriatric quality of life, geriatric population and improving their quality of life."] *Türk Geriatri Dergisi* 7(3):162–165.

[72] Başaran, Sibel, Rengin Güzel, and Tunay Sarpel. 2005. "Yaşam kalitesi ve sağlık sonuçlarını değerlendirme ölçütleri." ["Measures for the assessment of quality of life and health outcomes."]. *Romatizma* 20(1):55-63.

[73] Rabuş, Şule. 2007. *Diyabetik Hastalarda Tedavi Profilinin Belirlenmesi ve Topikal İnsulin Uygulanmasının Yara İyleşmesi Üzerine Etkilerinin İncelenmesi.* [*Identification of the Treatment Profile of the Patients with Diabetes and Assessment of the Effects of Topical Insulin Administration on Wound Healing.*]. PhD diss., Marmara University Institute of Health Sciences.

[74] Şenol, Yeşim, and Mehtap Türkay. 2006. "Yaşam kalitesi ölçütlerinde taraf tutma: cevap kayması." ["Bias at quality of life scales"]. *TAF Preventive Medicine Bulletin* 5(5):382-389.

[75] Shotorbani, Sudabe Azarmir. 2006. *Tüberküloz hastalarında yasam kalitesiölçülmesi ve silymarin'in antitüberküloz ilaç kaynaklı hepatotokisite üzerine etkisinin deneyhayvanlarında araştırılması.* [*Measurement of quality of life in tuberculosis patients and investigation of the effect of silymarin on antituberculous drug-induced hepatotoxicity in experimental animals*]. PhD diss., Marmara University Institute of Health Sciences.

[76] Juniper, Elizabeth F., A. Sonia Buist, Fred M. Cox, Penelope J. Ferrie, and Derek R. King. 1999. "Validation of a standardized version of the Asthma Quality of Life Questionnaire." *Chest* 115:1265-70.

[77] Blanco, Ignacio, Frederick J de Serres, Enrique Fernández-Bustillo, Beatriz Lara, and Marc Miravitlles. 2006. "Estimated numbers and prevalence of PI*S and PI*Z alleles of alpha1-antitrypsin deficiency in European countries." *Eur. Respir. J.* 27(1):77-84.

[78] Soydeğer, Başak. 2008. *Kronik Obstrüktif Akciğer Hastalığı Olan Hastalarda, İlaç Profilinin Belirlenmesi ve Hastaların Yaşam*

Kalitelerinin Değerlendirilmesi. [*Determination of the Medication Profile and Evaluation of Quality of Life of Patients with Chronic Obstructive Pulmonary Disease.*]. Msc diss., Marmara University Institute of Health Sciences.

[79] Jolicoeur, Lynn M., Amy J. Jones-Grizzle, and J. Gregory Boyer. 1992. "Guidelines for Performing a Pharmacoeconomic Analysis." *American Journal of Health-System Pharmacy* 49(7):1741-1747.

[80] Balık, Ali. 2008. *Gazi Hastanesi Çocuk Alerji ve Astım Bilimdalında Yeni Astım Tansı Konan Hastaların Tanı ve Tedavi Öncesi Yıllık Maliyeti* [*Annual Costs Before Receiving Diagnosis and Treatment of Asthma of the Patients with New Asthma Diagnosis at the Pediatric Allergy and Asthma Department of Gazi Hospital*]. Gazi Üniversitesi Tıp Fakültesi Çocuk Sağlığı ve Hastalıkları Anabilim Dalı.

[81] Juniper, Elizabeth F., Gordon H Guyatt, Andrew Willan, and Lauren L Griffith. 1994. "Determining a minimal important change in a disease-specific Quality of Life Questionnaire." *J Clin Epidemiol* 47:81-7.

[82] Juniper, Elizabeth F., Gordon H. Guyatt, Robert S. Epstein, Penelope J. Ferrie, Roman Jaeschke, and, TK Hiller. 1992. "Evaluation of impairment of health related quality of life in asthma: development of a questionnaire for use in clinical trials." *Thorax*, 47 (2): 76–83.

[83] GINA. 2011. "Global Strategy for Asthma Management and Prevention: 2011 Update." https://ginasthma.org/wp-content/uploads/2019/01/2011-GINA.pdf.

[84] Thomas, Mike, Stephen Kay, James Pike, Angela Williams, Jacqueline R Carranza Rosenzweig, Elizabeth V Hillyer, and David Price. 2009. "The Asthma Control Test (ACT) as a Predictor of GINA Guideline-Defined Asthma Control: Analysis of a Multinational Cross-Sectional Survey." *Primary Care Respiratory Journal* 18(1):41-49.

[85] Korenblat, Phillip E. 2001. "The Role of Antileukotrienes in the Treatment of Asthma." *Annals of Allergy, Asthma & Immunology* 86(6):31-39.

[86] Tohda, Y., M. Fujimura, H. Taniguchi, K. Takagi, T. Igarashi, H. Yasuhara, K. Takahashi, and S. Nakajima. 2002. "Leukotriene Receptor Antagonist, Montelukast can Reduce the Need for Inhaled Steroid while Maintaining the Clinical Stability of Asthmatic Patients." *Clinical Experimental Allergy* 32(8):1180-1186.

[87] Laviolette, Michel, Kerstin Malmstrom, Susan Lu, Paul Chervinsky, Jean-Claude Pujet, Izabella Peszek, Ji Zhang, and Theodore F. Reiss. 1999. "Montelukast Added to Inhaled Beclomethasone in Treatment of Asthma." *American Journal of Respiratory and Critical Care Medicine* 160(6):1862-1868.

[88] Coutts, Jonathan A, Neil A Gibson, and James Y Paton. 1992. "Measuring Compliance with Inhaled Medication in Asthma." *Archives of Disease in Childhood* 67(3):332-333.

[89] Strunk, Robert C., and Gordon R. Bloomberg. 2006. "Omalizumab for Asthma." *New England Journal of Medicine* 354(25):2689-2695.

[90] Zdanowicz, Martin M. 2007. "Pharmacotherapy of Asthma." *American Journal of Pharmaceutical Education* 71(5):98.

[91] Leuppi, Joerg D., Claudia Steurer-Stey, Manuela Peter, Prashant N. Chhajed, Johannes H. Wildhaber, and François Spertini. 2006. "Asthma Control in Switzerland: A General Practitioner Based Survey." *Current Medical Research and Opinion* 22(11):2159-2166.

[92] Laforest, Laurent, Eric Van Gasse, Gilles Devouassoux, Stephanie Chretin, Liesl M Osman, Gisele Bauguil, Yves Pacheco, and Genevieve Chamba. 2006. "Management of Asthma in Patients Supervised by Primary Care Physicians or by Specialists." *European Respiratory Journal* 27(1):42-50.

[93] Minoguchi, Kenji, Yasurou Kohno, Hideko Minoguchi, Norio Kihara, Yasuyuki Sano, Hajime Yasuhara, and Mitsuru Adachi. 2002. "Reduction of Eosinophilic Inflammation in the Airways of Patients with Asthma Using Montelukast." *Chest* 121(3):732-738.

[94] Calhoun, William J., Bernard J. Lavins, Margaret C. Minkwitz, Rhobert Evans, Gerald J. Gleich, and Judith Cohn. 1998. "Effect of Zafirlukast (Accolate) on Cellular Mediators of Inflammation." *American Journal of Respiratory and Critical Care Medicine* 157(5):1381-1389.

[95] Sampson, Anthony P., Emilio Pizzichini, and Hans Bisgaard. 2003. "Effects of Cysteinyl Leukotrienes and Leukotriene Receptor Antagonists on Markers of Inflammation." *Journal of Allergy and Clinical Immunology* 111(1):S49-S61.

[96] Ringdal, Nils, Avraham Eliraz, R. Pruzinec, Hans H. Weber, Paul G. H. Mulder, Martjin Akveld, and Eric D. Bateman. 2003. "The Salmeterol/Fluticasone Combination is More Effective than Fluticasone Plus Oral Montelukast in Asthma." *Respiratory Medicine* 97(3):234-241.

[97] Wilson, Andrew M., Owen J. Dempsey, Erika J. Sims, and Brian J. Lipworth. 2001. "Evaluation of Salmeterol or Montelukast as Second-Line Therapy for Asthma not Controlled with Inhaled Corticosteroids." *Chest* 119(4):1021-1026.

[98] Halbert, Ronald J., David G. Tinkelman, Denise R. Globe, and Shao-Lee Lin. 2009. "Measuring Asthma Control is the First Step to Patient Management: A Literature Review." *Journal of Asthma* 46(7):659-664.

[99] El Hasnaoui, Abdelkader, Jennifer Martin, Hocine Salhi, and Adam Doble. 2009. "**Validation of the Asthma Control Test Questionnaire in a North African Population.**" *Respiratory Medicine* 103:S30-S37.

[100] Virchow, Johann Christian, and Claus Bachert. 2006. "Efficacy and Safety of Montelukast in Adults with Asthma and Allergic Rhinitis." *Respiratory Medicine* 100(11):1952-1959.

[101] Samarzija, Miroslav, Marko Jakopovic, Fadila Pavicic, Suzana Kukulj, Sanja Popovic-Grle, and Zlata Beg-Zeg. 2005. "Montelukast in asthma treatment in Croatia." *Coll Antropoll* 29(2):683-8.

[102] Virchow, Johann Christian, Anish Mehta, Li Ljungblad, and Harald Mitfessel. 2010. "Add-On Montelukast in Inadequately Controlled Asthma Patients in a 6-Month Open-Label Study: The Montelukast

in Chronic Asthma (MONICA) Study." *Respiratory Medicine* 104(5):644-651.

[103] Chaudhury, Alisha, Gajanan S. Gaude, Jyothi Hattiholi. 2017. "Effects of oral montelukast on airway function in acute asthma: A randomized trial." *Lung India* 34(4):349-354.

[104] Zubairi, Ali Bin Sarwar, Nawal Salahuddin, Ali Khawaja, Safia Awan, Adil Ajiaz Shah, Ahmed Suleman Haque, Shahid Javed Husain, Nisar Rao, and Javaid Ahmad Khan AS. 2013. "A randomized, double-blind, placebo-controlled trial of oral montelukast in acute asthma exacerbation." *BMC Pulm Med* 13(1):20.

[105] Humbert, Marc, Stephen T. Holgate, Louis-Philippe Boulet, and Jean Bousquet. 2007. "Asthma Control or Severity: That is the Question." *Allergy* 62(2):95-101.

[106] Ullah Baig, Mirza Saif, Rashid Ahmed Khan, Kamran Khan, and Nadeem Rizvi. 2019. "Effectiveness and Quality of Life with Montelukast in Asthma – A Double-Blind Randomized Control Trial." *Pakistan Journal of Medical Sciences* 35(3):731-736.

[107] FitzGerald, J Mark, Sylvain Foucart, Stephen Coyle, John Sampalis, Denis Haine, Eliofotisti Psaradellis, and R Andrew McIvor. 2009. "Montelukast as Add-On Therapy to Inhaled Corticosteroids in the Management of Asthma (The SAS Trial)." *Canadian Respiratory Journal* 16(suppl a):5A-10A.

[108] Dupont, Lieven, Emmanuel Potvin, Dana Korn, Albert Lachman, Michèle Dramaix, Julie Gusman, and Rudi Peché. 2005. "Improving Asthma Control in Patients Suboptimally Controlled on Inhaled Steroids and Long-Acting B2- Agonists: Addition of Montelukast in an Open-Label Pilot Study." *Current Medical Research and Opinion* 21(6):863-869.

[109] Noonan, Michael J., Paul Chervinsky, Milan Brandon, Ji Zhang, Sayandeep Kundu, Jennifer McBurney, and Theodore F. Reiss. 1998. "Montelukast, A Potent Leukotriene Receptor Antagonist, Causes Dose-Related Improvements in Chronic Asthma." *European Respiratory Journal* 11(6):1232-1239.

[110] Şahin, Bayram, and Mehtap Tatar. 2006. "Factors Affecting Use of Resources for Asthma Patients." *Journal of Medical Systems* 30 (5): 395-403.

[111] Creticos, Peter S. 2003. "Treatment Options for Initial Maintenance Therapy of Persistent Asthma." *Drugs* 63(Supplement 2):1-20.

[112] Chen, Hubert, Michael K. Gould, Paul D. Blanc, Dave P. Miller, Tripthi V. Kamath, June H. Lee, and Sean D. Sullivan. 2007. "Asthma Control, Severity, and Quality of Life: Quantifying the Effect of Uncontrolled Disease." *Journal of Allergy and Clinical Immunology* 120(2):396-402.

[113] Chhabra, Sunil K., and Shivu Kaushik. 2005. "Validation of the asthma quality of life questionnaire (AQLQ-UK English Version) in Indian Asthmatic Subjects." *Indian J Chest Dis Allied Sci* 47:167-173.

In: The Pharmacological Guide to Montelukast ISBN: 978-1-53616-394-0
Editor: Søren C. Dam   © 2019 Nova Science Publishers, Inc.

Chapter 3

THE EFFICACY OF MONTELUKAST IN THE TREATMENT OF ALLERGIC RHINITIS

Cigdem Kalaycik Ertugay, MD and Ela Araz Server, MD

Department of Otorhinolaryngology/Head
and Neck Surgery Istanbul Education and Research Hospital,
Istanbul, Turkey

ABSTRACT

Leukotrienes, formed by leukocytes, are the inflammatory mediators which play an active role both in the early and late-phase immune response. Cysteinyl-leukotriene receptor antagonists are used in the treatment of allergic rhinitis as they inhibit the end-organ response by blocking the leukotriene receptors. This group includes montelukast, zafirlukast and prankulast. Montelukasts are effective on congestion, rhinorrhea, itching and sneezing which compromise the four main daytime symptoms of allergic rhinitis. Antihistaminics and nasal steroids are the main treatment modalities in allergic rhinitis. However, when compared with the placebo, montelukast is more effective on nasal and ocular symptoms. ARIA guideline also proposed montelukast in the seasonal allergic rhinitis of adults and perennial allergic rhinitis of children. Recent studies have mainly focused on combined use of montelukast and antihistaminics and reported that these combinations are as effective as nasal steroids. Further double-blind placebo controlled studies with large study population which evaluates the efficacy of montelukast and also the combined use of montelukasts and antihistaminics should be performed. These studies can provide wider use of montelukast in the treatment of allergic rhinitis.

Keywords: rhinitis, allergic, perennial, rhinitis, allergic, seasonal, montelukast, leukotriene antagonists

INTRODUCTION

Allergic rhinitis is one of the most commonly seen diseases which remarkably decreases the quality of life. Relieving the symptoms is the main goal of the treatment of allergic rhinitis and pharmacotherapy is effective on the management of symptoms by directly inhibiting the functions of the mediators of allergic reaction. Therefore, it is the primary treatment modality. In addition to antihistamines and steroids which have been widely used in the treatment, montelukasts also have recently been proposed in the literature. In order to understand the role of montelukasts in the treatment; the pathogenesis and the classification of allergic rhinitis should be mentioned.

ALLERGIC RHINITIS

Rhinitis is defined as the inflammation of the nasal mucosa. Allergic rhinitis, on the other hand, is considered as a subtype of rhinitis which results from the immune response of the human body and manifested with sneezing, nasal itching, nasal discharge and the obstruction of the nose [1]. It is commonly seen both in the pediatric and adult population. Although the prevalence of allergic rhinitis differs throughout the world, it is estimated to effect over 500 million people. It is accepted to be a serious health issue due to its negative effect on the quality of life together with its economic burden.

Allergic rhinitis is an immunoglobulin-E (Ig E) dependent type-1 hypersensitivity reaction. Activated Ig E triggers the antigen presentation, differentiation of T-cell, degranulation of the mast cell and the secretion of inflammatory mediators respectively. These mediators are responsible for the symptoms of the disease. They lead to two kinds of immune responses: early and late phase. In previously sensitized patients, early response is seen immediately after the antigen exposure and it lasts for 2-4 hours. Mast cell degranulation is the main component of the early phase response which leads to the release of histamine, prostaglandin, leukotriene, protease, proteoglycan, cytokine and chemokine. These mediators are responsible for the edema, for increased vascular permeability and the subsequent nasal discharge. Histamine is the main mediator of the early phase. Stimulation of the sensory fibers of the trigeminal nerve by histamine results in sneezing and itching. It also acts on the vessels together with leukotrienes and prostaglandins which leads to nasal congestion and nasal obstruction. Late phase response starts 4-6 hours after the antigen exposure. T-lymphocytes, basophils and eosinophils are the main actors in the late phase. They secrete leukotriene, kinin, histamine, chemokine and cytokine. Late phase is mainly related with nasal congestion [2].

The diagnosis of allergic rhinitis is dependent on the clinical manifestations. Therefore, its classification and treatment mainly rely on the symptoms. The time of antigen exposure, severity and the frequency of the symptoms are cardinal steps for the classification. Depending on the time of antigen exposure, it is subdivided into four groups:

- Seasonal allergic rhinitis: Symptoms occur during the same season of the year, when the patient is exposed to the antigen.
- Perennial allergic rhinitis: Symptoms occur throughout the year.
- Acute intermittent (episodic) allergic rhinitis: Symptoms occur in random episodes (in sensitized patients) throughout the year.

- Seasonal episodes of the chronic disease: Symptoms occur throughout the year with episodic aggravations.

This classification has been used in the clinical practice but it still couldn't cover a group of patients whose manifestations were challenging to manage. Relying on this fact, World Health Organization (WHO) announced a new classification in 2001 titled as 'Allergic Rhinitis and its Impact on Asthma (ARIA).' When compared with the previous classification, ARIA introduced the terms 'intermittent' and 'persistent' instead of 'seasonal' and 'perennial.' The severity of the disease (mild, moderate, severe) is also integrated [1].

Allergic rhinitis triggers both local and systemic inflammatory responses by affecting the upper and lower respiratory tract. Therefore, additional comorbidities could be seen following the inflammation of the nasal mucosa. Asthma, rhino-sinusitis and conjunctivitis are the most commonly seen comorbidities. Coexistence of asthma and allergic rhinitis plays an important role in the management process. Although these two disorders effect the different parts of the respiratory tract and are considered as separate clinical issues, their overlapping etiopathogenic factors favor a common treatment approach. Both the upper and the lower respiratory tract share similar anatomic, physiologic, pathogenic and immunologic properties. They have a common lymphatic drainage. Therefore, a recent concept of 'Single Airway Disease' has been accepted [3]. Asthma should always be taken into consideration during the management of allergic rhinitis and it takes part in the ARIA guideline.

The symptoms of allergic rhinitis could be controlled by a proper diagnostic and management process. The main goal of the treatment is to increase the quality of life by relieving the symptoms. The first step includes the identification of the allergen and the prevention of exposure by eliminating the environmental factors. Prevention of the exposure may decrease the severity of the allergic response but cannot completely suppress the inflammatory reaction. In order to overcome the symptoms of the disease, medical treatment is commonly needed [4].

Inflammatory mediators are responsible for the symptoms of allergic rhinitis. Medical treatment aims to relieve the symptoms by blocking the functions of the mediators despite the fact that it has no effect on the natural course of the disease. Immunotherapy is the only treatment modality which both alters the course of the disease and relieves the symptoms. Although immunotherapy is the most convenient treatment modality, pharmacotherapy is still being used more commonly. There are many drugs of choices and the main step of the treatment includes the proper combinations of these drugs specifically for each patient. Recently, the treatment protocol of ARIA has been widely accepted [5].

Oral antihistamines occupy the first choice of treatment as they block the histamine which plays the most important role in the pathophysiologic process. Intranasal steroids are considered to be the second choice due to their strong effects on the symptoms. In moderate and severe allergic rhinitis, intranasal steroids are reported to be effective on sneezing, itching, nasal obstruction, nasal discharge and the ocular symptoms [5, 6]. ARIA also suggests anti-leukotrienes as an alternative choice depending on the recent studies which considered the effects of anti-leukotrienes on the symptoms of allergic rhinitis and comorbid diseases.

ANTILEUKOTRIENES

Leukotrienes (LT) are the inflammatory mediators which are secreted by leukocytes. They are contributed both in the early and the late phase of the disease [7]. LTC4, LTD4 and LTE4 are called cystenil leukotrienes and their functions include the contraction of the muscles of the bronchi, secretion of the mucus, increment of the vascular permeability and the production of subsequent edema. LTD4 enhances the nasal blood flow leading to nasal congestion. Anti-leukotrienes diminish the effects of these mediators and are subdivided into two groups: Cystenil leukotriene receptor antagonists (LTRA) interfere with the end organ response by blocking the leukotriene receptors. This group of agents include montelukast, zafirlukast and pranlukast. Leukotriene synthesis inhibitors inhibit the synthesis of cystenil leukotrienes and LTB4. This group includes zileuton, ZD-2138, Bay X 1005 and MK-0591. Montelukast is approved by FDA and is the most commonly used drug in the treatment of allergic rhinitis [7, 8].

MONTELUKAST AND ALLERGIC RHINITIS

Montelukast is effective on the four cardinal symptoms of allergic rhinitis which are congestion, rhinorrhea, itching and sneezing [7]. There are many studies focusing on the effect of montelukast on allergic rhinitis. Meta-analysis of these studies suggested the remarkable effect of montelukast both on the symptoms and the quality of life when compared with the placebo. However, they are reported to be less effective when compared with the antihistamines and intranasal steroids [9, 10, 11, 12]. The clinical effect of montelukast depends on the classification of the disease, the age of the patient and the presence or absence of any comorbidities. Studies reported that montelukasts are more effective on seasonal allergic rhinitis. In case of seasonal allergic rhinitis, when compared with the placebo, leukotriene receptor antagonists increase the quality of life by relieving daily nasal and ocular symptoms and are as effective as oral H1 antihistamines. However, they are less effective when compared with intranasal steroids [9, 10]. Although both LTRA and antihistamines have similar effects on allergic rhinitis, antihistamines are found to be more effective on daytime nasal and ocular symptoms whereas LTRA have stronger effect on nighttime symptoms such as difficulty falling asleep, arousals and awakening with a congested nose [12].

Regarding the age of the patient, montelukasts are more effective in pediatric seasonal allergic rhinitis and in adult perennial allergic rhinitis [6]. In case of any comorbidities, they diminish both the symptoms of rhinitis and asthma which is mainly provoked by the exercise and aspirin and are more effective when compared with oral antihistamines [13, 14]. LTRAs could be used for nasal symptoms of chronic sinusitis with nasal polyps but they have similar effects with intranasal steroids. Therefore, additional LTRA treatment is not recommended [15].

The latest version of ARIA (2016) guideline suggests both montelukasts and oral antihistamines as the first choice of treatment for seasonal allergic rhinitis. On the other hand, oral antihistamines are reported to be the main step in perennial allergic rhinitis [14]. It is also emphasized that the antihistamines are found to be more cost effective.

Montelukasts contribute an important role both as a single or as a part of a combination therapy. The combination of leukotriene antagonists and antihistamines are reported to be more effective on nasal discharge, itching, sneezing and daytime symptoms when compared with oral antihistamines alone [16]. Desloratadine - montelukast combination has a stronger effect on the symptoms of intermittent or mild persistent allergic rhinitis. In case of coexisting asthma, combination of these two agents in the same pharmaceutical agent increases the patient compliance and is considered to be more cost effective [17]. When antihistamines alone are not satisfactory, montelukast could be recommended in the second step.

In conclusion, montelukasts are remarkably effective agents on seasonal allergic rhinitis. In terms of cost effectiveness, although oral antihistamines are mainly preferred, montelukasts could be preferred as an alternative or additional treatment modality.

REFERENCES

[1]   Bousquet J, Van Cauwenberge P, Khaltaev N; Aria Workshop Group; World Health Organization. 2001. 'Allergic rhinitis and its impact on asthma.' *J Allergy Clin Immunol* 108:147–334. PMID: 11707753.

[2]   Pawankar R, Hayashi M, Yamanishi S, Igarashi T. 2015. 'The paradigm of cytokine networks in allergic airway inammation.' *Curr Opin Allergy Clin Immunol* 15:41-48. doi: 10.1097/ACI.0000000000000129.

[3] Braunstahl GJ. 2009. 'United airways concept: what does it teach us about systemic in ammation in airways disease?' *Proc Am Thorac Soc.* 6:652–4. doi: 10.1513/pats.200906-052DP.

[4] Matsui EC, Abramson SL, Sandel MT. 2016 'Indoor Environmental Control Practices and Asthma Management.' *Pediatrics.* 138(5). doi:10.1542/peds.2016-2589.

[5] Bousquet J, Khaltaev N, Cruz AA, Denburg J, Fokkens WJ, Togias A, et al. 2008. 'Allergic Rhinitis and its Impact on Asthma (ARIA)2008 update (in collaboration with the World Health Organization, GA2LEN and AllerGen).' *Allergy* 63: 86: 8-160. doi:10.1111/j.1398-9995.2007.01620.x.

[6] Seidman MD, Gurgel RK, Lin SY, Schwartz SR, Baroody FM, Bonner JR, et al. 2005.'Clinical practice guideline: Allergic rhinitis; Guideline Otolaryngology Development Group. AAO-HNSF.' *Otolaryngol Head Neck Surg.* 152(1 Suppl):S1-43. (doi:10.1177/0194599814561600).

[7] Cobanoğlu B, Toskala E, Ural A, Cingi C. 2013. 'Role of leukotriene antagonists and antihistamines in the treatment.' *Curt Allergy Asthma Rep* 13(2):203-8. doi: 10.1007/s11882-013-0341-4.

[8] Peters-Golden M, Henderson WR Jr. 2005. 'The role of leukotrienes in allergic rhinitis.' *Ann Allergy Asthma Immunol.* 94(6):609-18; quiz 618-20, 669. doi: 10.1016/S1081-1206(10)61317-8.

[9] Wilson AM, O'Byrne PM, Parameswaran K. 2004 'Leukotriene receptor antagonists for allergic rhinitis: a systematic review and meta-analysis.' *Am J Med* 116(5):338-44. doi: 10.1016/j.amjmed.2003.10.030.

[10] Rodrigo GJ, Yanez A. 2006. 'The role of antileukotriene therapy in seasonal allergic rhinitis: A systematic review of randomized trials.' *Ann Allergy Asthma Immunol* 96:779-86. doi: 10.1016/S1081-1206(10)61339-7.

[11] Grainger J, Drake-Lee A. 2006. 'Montelukast in allergic rhinitis: a systematic review and metaanalysis.' *Clin Otolaryngol* 31(5):360-7. doi:10.1111/j.1749-4486.2006.01276.x.

[12] Xu Y, Zhang J, Wang J. 2014. 'The efficacy and safety of selective H1-antihistamine versus leukotriene receptor antagonist for seasonal allergic rhinitis: a meta analysis.' *PLoS One* 9(11):e112815. doi:10.1371/journal.pone.0112815. 383622.

[13] Philip G, Nayak AS, Berger WE, Leynadier F, Vrijens F, Dass SB, et al. 2004. 'The effect of montelukast on rhinitis symptoms in patients with asthma and seasonal allergic rhinitis.' *Curr Med Res Opin* 20(10):1549-58. doi: 10.1185/030079904X3348.

[14] Brożek JL, Bousquet J, Agache I, Agarwal A, Bachert C, Bosnic-Anticevich S et al. 2017. 'Allergic Rhinitis and its Impact on Asthma (ARIA) guidelines-2016 revision.' *J Allergy Clin Immunol.* Oct;140(4):950-958. doi: 10.1016/j. jaci.2017.03.050.

[15] Rudmik L, Soler ZM. 2015. 'Medical Therapies for Adult Chronic Sinusitis: A Systematic Review.' *JAMA* 314(9):926-39. doi: 10.1001/jama.2015.7544.

[16] Liu G, Zhou X, Chen J, Liu F. 2018. 'Oral Antihistamines Alone vs in Combination with Leukotriene Receptor Antagonists for Allergic Rhinitis: A Meta-analysis.' *Otolaryngol Head Neck Surg.* 158(3):450-458. doi:10.1177/0194599817752624.

[17] Cingi C, Oghan F, Eskiizmir G, Yaz A, Ural A, Erdogmus N. 2013. 'Desloratadine-montelukast combination improves quality of life and decreases nasal obstruction in patients with perennial allergic rhinitis.' *Int Forum Allergy Rhinol.* 3(10):801-6. doi: 10.1002/alr.21185.

INDEX

α

α-CD, 7, 9

β

β-CD, 7, 9, 10
Beta-2 Agonists, 41

γ

γ-CD, 7, 9

A

acute asthma, 71, 87
adolescents, 37, 48
adults, ix, 5, 15, 22, 23, 37, 38, 49, 89
adverse effects, 30, 33, 36, 37, 38, 42, 43, 44, 50, 52
age, viii, 4, 15, 20, 21, 23, 24, 26, 27, 31, 43, 44, 53, 55, 72, 94
agonist, viii, 20, 28, 31, 32, 33, 37, 40, 60, 61, 71
airway inflammation, 21, 25, 39, 70
airways, 23, 24, 25, 36, 39, 44, 96
allergens, 24, 25, 27, 29, 30, 38, 41, 45, 82
allergic, v, vii, ix, 1, 3, 10, 14, 23, 24, 29, 38, 40, 43, 45, 77, 86, 89, 90, 91, 92, 93, 94, 95, 96, 97
allergic reaction, 23, 90
allergic rhinitis, ix, 3, 10, 29, 38, 40, 89, 90, 91, 92, 93, 94, 95, 96, 97
allergy, 11, 40, 58
anaphylaxis, 5, 39
antihistamines, 90, 93, 94, 95, 96
anti-lgE, 43
arrhythmia, 42, 44
assessment, 21, 29, 46, 47, 48, 54, 83
asthma, v, vii, viii, 1, 2, 6, 9, 10, 11, 14, 15, 17, 18, 19, 20, 21, 22, 23, 24, 25, 26, 27, 28, 29, 30, 31, 32, 33, 34, 35, 36, 37, 38, 39, 40, 41, 43, 44, 45, 46, 48, 49, 50, 51, 52, 53, 54, 57, 58, 59, 60, 61, 62, 63, 64, 66, 67, 68, 69, 70, 71, 72, 73, 74, 75, 76, 77, 78, 79, 80, 81, 82, 83, 84, 85, 86, 87, 88, 92, 94, 95, 96, 97
asthma attacks, 30, 43, 71
asthma control, viii, 20, 22, 32, 33, 34, 35, 36, 39, 48, 52, 53, 54, 61, 62, 63, 64, 66, 67, 69, 70, 72, 74, 78, 79, 80, 81, 84, 85, 86, 87, 88

Index

Asthma Control Test (ACT), viii, 20, 22, 34, 35, 53, 54, 61, 62, 63, 64, 66, 67, 68, 69, 70, 71, 72, 74, 78, 80, 84, 86
Asthma Quality of Life Questionnaire (AQLQ), viii, 20, 22, 34, 48, 49, 53, 54, 65, 66, 67, 68, 73, 74, 83, 88
atopic dermatitis, 3, 28, 58
atopy, 23, 24, 29, 58

B

basophils, 25, 39, 91
bile, 5, 40
bioavailability, vii, 2, 6, 7, 10, 14, 16, 39, 40
blood, 5, 11, 13, 33, 42, 70, 93
breathing, 28, 50
bronchoconstriction, 25, 31, 39
bronchodilator, viii, 20, 22, 27, 28, 29, 32, 33, 39, 42, 70
bronchospasm, 36, 40, 43

C

calcium, 10, 12
candidiasis, 38, 61
capsule, 10, 11, 17
CDC, 21, 75
chemical, 10, 12
chewable tablets, 4
childhood, 24, 46, 56, 57, 82
children, ix, 4, 15, 21, 22, 23, 26, 27, 37, 40, 44, 48, 65, 89
chitosan nanoparticles, 6, 15
chromones, 43
chronic diseases, viii, 20, 21, 50
chronotherapeutic oral dosage form, 11
cigarette smoke, 27, 50
classification, 35, 54, 55, 90, 91, 92, 94
classification of asthma severity, 31
clinical application, 12, 13, 49
clinical trials, 14, 49, 84

combination therapy, 69, 95
commercial, 9, 11, 17, 55
compliance, 10, 44, 52, 95
composition, 9, 13, 17
controlled studies, ix, 70, 90
COPD, 29, 76, 81, 82
coronary arteries, 11, 13
coronary artery disease, 57, 58
correlation, 34, 38, 40, 55, 64, 67, 68, 71, 74
corticosteroids, 5, 29, 30, 32, 36, 37, 40, 60, 68, 69, 70, 71, 72
cost, 12, 21, 95
cough, 21, 23, 27, 33, 39, 46, 50, 51, 60
cyclodextrins, viii, 2, 7, 8, 9, 10, 16
cytochrome, 5, 43
cytokines, 24, 26

D

definition, 22, 47
derivatives, 7, 9, 42
diabetes, 48, 57, 83
diagnosis, 27, 28, 29, 35, 46, 50, 75, 76, 77, 79, 81, 82, 84, 91
diseases, 14, 24, 25, 28, 29, 48, 49, 72, 90, 93
distress, 21, 49
dosage, vii, 1, 2, 4, 6, 8, 10, 11, 12, 30, 44
drainage, 92
drug delivery, 2, 11, 15, 16, 17
drug dosage forms, 2
drugs, 5, 9, 12, 21, 30, 35, 39, 42, 70, 93

E

eczema, 28, 58
edema, 5, 15, 25, 58, 91, 93
education, 22, 30, 44, 51
emergency, 21, 44
encapsulation, viii, 2, 5, 7, 8, 11, 12, 13
endothelial cells, 12, 13

energy, 7, 47
entothelial vascular cells, 12
environment, 26, 27, 45, 47
environmental factors, 21, 24, 25, 92
eosinophil, 24, 39, 70
eosinophil count, 24, 70
eosinophilia, 33, 34, 40
eosinophils, 23, 25, 26, 39, 70, 91
epidemiology, 23, 76, 77
exercise, 29, 31, 33, 41, 43, 51, 74, 94
expenditures, 23, 56
exposure, 21, 23, 25, 27, 38, 43, 46, 50, 55, 65, 66, 67, 68, 73, 91, 92

F

food, 5, 7, 16, 40, 60
Food and Drug Administration (FDA), 2, 6, 7, 9, 94
formation, 3, 9, 10
fragments, 7, 9

G

gastroesophageal reflux, 30, 60, 72
genetic factors, 21, 25
genetic predisposition, 25, 26
Global Initiative for Asthma (GINA), viii, 20, 22, 30, 35, 37, 53, 54, 61, 62, 63, 64, 66, 67, 69, 70, 74, 76, 77, 78, 84
glucocorticoids, 36
granules, 4, 8, 10, 15, 17
guidelines, viii, 20, 22, 33, 35, 53, 61, 62, 63, 64, 66, 67, 97

H

half-life, 5, 39
happiness, 47, 49
headache, 5, 42

health, 24, 48, 49, 50, 51, 56, 83, 84, 91
health care, 24, 51
histamine, 9, 10, 24, 25, 29, 38, 91, 93
history, 26, 27, 33, 34, 37, 46, 57, 58
homes, 56, 57
house dust, 27, 45
HPβCD, 7, 8, 9, 10
human, 7, 10, 12, 39, 43, 90
humidity, vii, 2, 4
hydroxybutenyl cyclodextrins, 9
hypersensitivity, 5, 33, 91
hypertrophy, 25, 26

I

ICS, viii, 20, 30, 32, 37, 60, 61
identification, 51, 52, 92
immune response, vii, ix, 89, 90, 91
immunoglobulin, 24, 43, 91
improvements, ix, 20, 69, 71, 72, 73
in vitro, 8, 12, 16, 17, 29
in vivo, 6, 9, 12, 16, 17, 29
incidence, 5, 23, 24
independent variable, 66, 67
individuals, 27, 28, 29, 47
infants, 5, 44
inflammation, 3, 12, 21, 23, 24, 25, 30, 70, 90, 92
inflammatory cells, 24, 26, 41
inflammatory mediators, vii, ix, 89, 91, 93
ingredients, 9, 10
inhaled steroids, 36, 37, 38, 43, 74, 87
inhaler, 37, 44, 52, 63, 72
inhibitor, 17, 22, 39
interactions, 5, 7, 9, 26
ipratropium bromide, 43

L

lactic acid, 2, 6
leukocytes, vii, ix, 89, 93

leukotriene antagonists, 36, 90, 95, 96
leukotriene modifier, vii, 1, 2
leukotriene modifying medications, 38
leukotriene receptor antagonists, ix, 22, 30, 39, 53, 69, 70, 73, 76, 86, 89, 93, 94, 97
leukotrienes, vii, 3, 14, 18, 24, 38, 91, 93, 96
light, vii, 2, 4, 14
Likert scale, 49, 54, 55
lipids, 6, 7
liver, 5, 39, 40
lymphocytes, 23, 24, 25, 26, 91

M

magnetic nanoparticles, 12
majority, 56, 57, 58, 71
management, vii, 1, 11, 15, 30, 36, 38, 90, 92
mast cells, 25, 39, 41
measurements, 21, 29, 46, 48, 64
mechanisms of asthma, 24
median, ix, 20, 62, 64
medical, 28, 48, 51, 92
medication, viii, 20, 22, 29, 32, 34, 36, 37, 43, 44, 50, 51, 53, 63
metabolism, 5, 14, 15, 43
metabolized, 39, 43
meter, 29, 30, 51
methylxanthines, 42
microparticles, 2
molecules, 2, 7, 9
montelukast, v, vii, viii, ix, 1, 2, 3, 4, 5, 6, 7, 8, 9, 10, 11, 12, 13, 14, 15, 16, 17, 18, 19, 20, 22, 38, 39, 40, 53, 61, 62, 63, 64, 65, 68, 69, 70, 71, 72, 73, 74, 76, 85, 86, 87, 89, 90, 93, 94, 95, 96, 97
morbidity, 21, 23, 24, 50
mortality, 21, 23, 24, 36, 50
mortality rate, 23, 24, 50
mucosa, viii, 2, 13, 25, 26, 38, 90, 92

mucus, 3, 25, 39, 41, 59, 93
muscles, 28, 42, 93

N

nanoemulsion, 8, 12, 16
nanoparticles, 2, 6, 7, 11, 13, 15, 18
nanostructured lipid carriers, 7, 16
nasal polyp, 27, 95
native cyclodextrins, 7, 9
nausea, 42, 61
nebulizer, 44, 52, 63
New England, 77, 81, 85
New Zealand, 23, 75
nitric oxide, 24, 33
nocturnal asthma, 11, 17

O

obstruction, 25, 28, 36, 90, 91, 93, 97
oral granules, 4, 15
organ, ix, 89, 93
outpatient, viii, 20, 21, 52

P

pain, 42, 48, 61, 63
pathogenesis, 25, 26, 78, 90
patient education, 30, 44, 51
patient history, 27
peak expiratory flow rate, 29, 71
perennial, ix, 89, 90, 91, 92, 94, 95, 97
permeability, 39, 41, 91, 93
pharmaceutical, 4, 7, 52, 95
pharmacological treatment, 49, 52
pharmacotherapy, 90, 93
physical examination, 27, 28
physicians, 34, 70
placebo, ix, 69, 70, 73, 74, 87, 89, 94
plasma proteins, 39, 40

Index

pollen, 27, 45
pollution, 24, 27, 46, 50, 60, 72
poly-lactic acid, 2, 6
polymer, 6, 9, 11
positive correlation, 70, 74
pranlukast, 39, 93
preparation, iv, 8, 17
prevention, 18, 31, 39, 45, 92
prophylactic, 40, 69
prostaglandin, 24, 26, 91
pulmonary function test, 28, 30, 33, 35, 70

Q

quality of life, v, vii, viii, 19, 20, 21, 22, 24, 36, 47, 48, 49, 50, 51, 53, 54, 55, 65, 66, 67, 69, 72, 73, 74, 75, 79, 83, 84, 87, 88, 90, 91, 92, 94, 97
questionnaire, 34, 49, 50, 54, 65, 70, 73, 84, 88

R

reactions, 3, 5, 37, 42
receptor, viii, ix, 2, 3, 14, 18, 20, 22, 30, 37, 38, 39, 40, 43, 53, 68, 69, 70, 73, 89, 93, 94, 96, 97
recommendations, iv, 4, 40
regression, 55, 66, 67
regression analysis, 55, 66
relatives, 57, 65
relief, 22, 70
requirement, 33, 72
response, ix, 11, 23, 24, 27, 28, 37, 43, 46, 49, 70, 89, 91, 92, 93
restenosis, 11, 18
rhinitis, v, ix, 3, 10, 29, 38, 40, 58, 78, 86, 89, 90, 91, 92, 93, 94, 95, 96, 97
rhinorrhea, ix, 38, 89, 94
risk, 21, 23, 26, 27, 29, 34, 37, 42, 46, 52, 59, 60

risk factors, 21, 23, 26, 27, 45, 52, 59, 60, 78
routes, 6, 12, 36, 44

S

safety, 14, 15, 97
seasonal, ix, 3, 89, 90, 91, 92, 94, 95, 96, 97
secretion, 24, 27, 39, 41, 91, 93
sensitivity, vii, 2, 28, 29, 45
serum, 40, 42, 43
severe asthma, 31, 39
shortness of breath, 22, 27, 33, 49, 50, 58, 63
sibling, 26, 27
sinusitis, 58, 92, 94
skin, 3, 29
smoking, 24, 46, 51, 52, 56, 57, 71
smooth muscle, 13, 25, 26, 41, 42
society, 21, 23
sodium, 3, 4, 8, 10, 14, 15, 16, 17, 36, 43
solid dosage forms, vii, 1, 4, 10
solid lipid nanoparticles, 7, 16
solubility, 3, 10
solution, 8, 14, 16
spirometry, 28, 29, 46, 64
sputum, 33, 34, 46, 70
stability, vii, 2, 6, 8, 9, 10, 14, 17
stabilization, 10, 12
stabilizers, 8, 9
standard deviation, 55, 61, 62, 64
starch, 10, 16
state, 23, 47
stent, 11, 18
steroids, ix, 36, 37, 38, 42, 43, 69, 74, 89, 90, 93, 94, 95
stimulation, 24, 26
stoves, 46, 56
swelling, 27, 58
symptom control, v, vii, viii, 19, 20, 22, 31, 69

symptoms, ix, 21, 22, 25, 27, 29, 30, 32, 33, 34, 35, 36, 37, 38, 39, 42, 43, 45, 49, 50, 51, 54, 55, 58, 59, 63, 65, 68, 70, 71, 73, 74, 89, 90, 91, 92, 93, 94, 95, 97
synthesis, 22, 26, 39, 93

T

target, 10, 11
targeted delivery, viii, 2, 12
techniques, viii, 2, 44, 51
therapy, 37, 39, 40, 43, 53, 68, 69, 71, 72, 73, 96
toxicity, 6, 42
treatment, v, vii, viii, ix, 5, 9, 10, 11, 14, 17, 19, 20, 21, 22, 24, 27, 30, 32, 33, 35, 36, 37, 39, 40, 42, 43, 44, 45, 46, 47, 48, 49, 50, 51, 52, 60, 61, 62, 63, 64, 69, 70, 71, 72, 73, 74, 75, 76, 77, 79, 81, 82, 83, 84, 85, 86, 88, 89, 90, 91, 92, 93, 94, 95, 96
trial, 71, 73, 87
triggers, 91, 92
tuberculosis, 57, 83
Turkey, 19, 23, 24, 52, 76, 77, 79, 89

V

variables, 21, 55
viral infection, 26, 60

W

water, 3, 4, 8, 9, 10, 41
weight gain, 5, 61
wheezing, 21, 22, 27, 28, 33, 50, 63
wood, 45, 56
World Health Organization (WHO), 24, 47, 48, 92, 95, 96
worldwide, 23, 24

Z

zafirlukast, vii, ix, 22, 38, 39, 70, 74, 86, 89, 93

Antibiotic Resistance: Causes and Risk Factors, Mechanisms and Alternatives

Editors: Adriel R. Bonilla and Kaden P. Muniz

Series: Pharmacology - Research, Safety Testing and Regulation

Book Description: This book addresses the concern that over the past few years, there has been a major rise in resistance to antibiotics among gram-negative bacteria. New antibacterial drugs with novel modes of actions are urgently required in order to fight against infection.

Hardcover ISBN: 978-1-60741-623-4
Retail Price: $265

Medicinal Plants and Sustainable Development

Editor: Chandra Prakash Kala (Indian Institute of Forest Management, Madhya Pradesh, India)

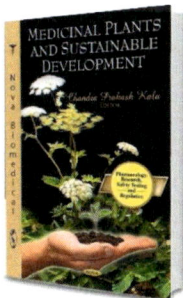

Series: Pharmacology - Research, Safety Testing and Regulation

Book Description: This book deals with multidisciplinary approach and contains information on different aspects of medicinal plants, which can be used as guiding tools.

Hardcover ISBN: 978-1-61761-942-7
Retail Price: $139

Pharmaceutical Innovation: Challenges and Competitors

Editors: Tomas E. Sanchez and Charles L. Scott

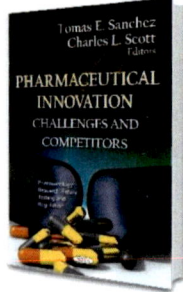

Series: Pharmacology - Research, Safety Testing and Regulation

Book Description: This book examines the challenges associated with striking the proper balance between lower cost drugs and maintaining an innovative domestic pharmaceutical sector.

Hardcover ISBN: 978-1-62257-068-3
Retail Price: $130

Human Serum Albumin (HSA): Functional Structure, Synthesis and Therapeutic Uses

Editor: Travis Stokes

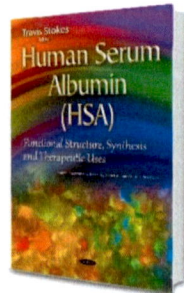

Series: Protein Biochemistry, Synthesis, Structure and Cellular Functions

Book Description: This book provides an overview of the expanding field of preclinical and clinical applications and developments that use albumin as a carrier of drug delivery systems.

Hardcover ISBN: 978-1-63482-963-2
Retail Price: $230